Plant-Based Di

Complete St   Guide for:
Cooking Healthy Dishes, Restore
your Workout and Always Have the
Right Amount of Energy

Annie T. Jenkins

a licensed professional before attempting any techniques outlined in this book.

By reading this document, the reader agrees that under no circumstances is the author responsible for any losses, direct or indirect, that are incurred as a result of the use of the information contained within this document, including, but not limited to, errors, omissions, or inaccuracies.

Table of Contents

Introduction

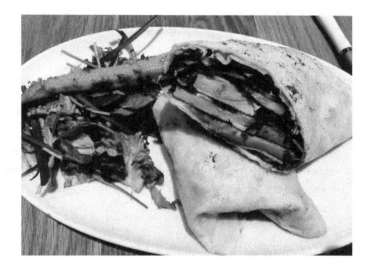

Athletes today are eating better than ever before. They are continuously consulting with dieticians, personal trainers, and medical professionals about what works best for their lifestyle. There are specific nutrients that play an important role in the development of muscle tissue and bone strength, as well as weight loss and increased energy. During this process, there have been many diets focusing on new and improved ways to build a leaner, stronger, and more efficient body type for superior athletic performance. Diets and eating lifestyles such as paleo, ketogenic, intermittent fasting and other diets have all shown some measure of promise and results. While there is success to varying degrees with many different diets and ways of eating, the vegan or plant-based diet is the best way.

There are a lot of myths about eating vegan in connection with a physically active lifestyle. For many years, there were myths and inaccuracies believed about plant-based eating and living which, fortunately, have been proven wrong. Indeed, new evidence provides far more research and findings to support the benefits of a vegan diet. It's important to learn what these myths are, versus their accurate findings, before incorporating a plant-based diet into your lifestyle.

What are some of the myths about plant-based eating and physical activity for athletes?

1. Athletes need lots of protein and these levels can only be found in red meat. While it is accurate that high levels of protein are contained in red meat, it does not mean you must eat it for this purpose. In fact, there are more sources of protein found in plants than meat which provide all the required amino acids for our body. B12 is another nutrient that is believed to only be found in red meat, though it can also be found in sources such as fermented soy (tempeh, miso) and brewer's yeast.

2. There is not enough iron and minerals in a vegan diet. Fortunately, this is untrue, as there are many

sources of all nutrients in vegetables, fruits, nuts, seeds, and other plant-based foods. In fact, there are more nutrients, including proteins and calcium in vegan food options, which are better absorbed and used by the body than meat-based proteins. All nine amino acids needed by our bodies can be found within a vegan diet; our body requires twenty amino acids in total, eleven of which we produce on our own, and nine we require in our diet.

3. Some people believe that dairy is required to achieve the required amount of calcium in your diet. While milk, yogurt, and cheese provide this nutrient, dairy is not the only option for calcium. Dark leafy greens, grains, and other vegetables can provide enough for your daily needs without having to consume any animal-based products at all.

4. Due to the myth that vegans need to have animal products in their diet to thrive and avoid deficiency, it's often expected that supplements are a must, without exception, and while many plant-based diets support supplements, it's not necessary to include them if you cover all of your daily requirements in the food choices you eat. Diets including meat and dairy, if not well balanced, can lead to a number of deficiencies, which prompts people to take supplements, even if they have access to all the nutrients they need in their food. This myth is widely taken out of proportion.

5. A lot of people still think of plant-based diets as boring and a fad, when in reality, veganism has been around for centuries and is a part of many cultures and eating habits worldwide. The variety of meals,

recipes, and food options are unlimited because vegan options include all vegetables, fruits, and other plant-based foods that you can combine to produce many dishes for all occasions. Spices, seasonings and the various pungent flavors of onions, shallots, and other strong-tasting foods add a lot of dimension to the meals that can be created.

6. Another myth about vegan diets and athletes, specifically bodybuilders, is the misperception of limited muscle growth, which is believed to be due to a lack of animal-based nutrients. This has been proven inaccurate, especially with the rise of vegan athletes, including Olympic competitors.

Veganism is on the rise in many societies and more people of all backgrounds are giving plant-based eating an honest try. Some reasons for this change in lifestyle and diet go beyond health and weight loss. For some, living a plant-based lifestyle means taking a proactive approach towards environmentalism and compassion for animals, while others adopt the lifestyle because of religious or spiritual reasons. The purpose of this book is to help support you as you explore this lifestyle by providing a step-by-step guide to incorporating veganism into your life. The goal is to empower you to enhance and improve your athletic lifestyle and to help you gain all the benefits that occur as a result.

Chapter 1: What Is a Plant-based Diet?

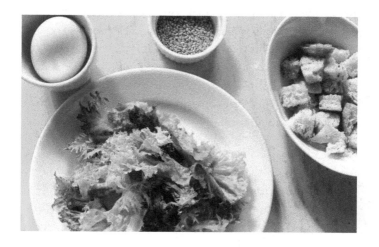

A plant-based diet is a popular and healthy way to eat for a good portion of the world's population. It includes a diet where all food choices are made from plant sources, and any animal-based foods such as meat and dairy are eliminated completely. Veganism is another term for plant-based eating. When adapting to this way of eating, it can take some people longer than others. There are stages between a regular diet with dairy and meat to veganism, and these can be implemented in steps where certain foods are reduced or minimized over time, such as specific meats (i.e. pork and beef). At the same time, vegetables, fruits, and other plant-based foods are increased.

Veganism can also be a philosophy, and many people eliminate animal-based foods and products from their lifestyle as a way to reject using animals. For many people, plant-based eating is a diet on the surface, while the commitment to abstaining from animal products extends much further. This may include abstaining from leather, fur, and other animal-based products used in clothing, makeup, and other household items. Veganism is synonymous with the animal rights' movement and strives to encourage people to avoid all forms of animal use in the products they consume.

Veganism is on the rise in many parts of the world due to its health benefits and sustainability. For many people in developing countries, beans, rice, and legumes are the central part of their cuisine, and while meat is often included as well, a diet largely comprised of vegetables and plant-based options is an excellent way to prevent many diseases and chronic conditions, as well as to provide relief to people who suffer from them. Overall, plant-based eating is a simple strategy for a better way of life and eating.

What Are the Benefits of a Plant-based Diet?

There are plenty of benefits associated with adopting a plant-based diet. Some people experience the positive effects of veganism earlier in the process, while others notice the advantages over a longer time frame. The benefits are common and unfold as your body becomes accustomed to the dietary changes.

- Weight loss is one of the major advantages of eating more vegetables and plant-based foods because they contain high amounts of fiber, which increases your metabolic function. Studies indicate that vegans have a lower body mass index and generally tend to be slimmer. This is largely due to the high level of fiber in vegetables and fruits, which make up a major part of the diet. Fiber helps your body process and absorb nutrients more quickly and efficiently than omnivorous or meat-based diets.

- A plant-based diet reduces your risk of cardiovascular disease. If heart conditions run in your family as an increased genetic risk, you can reduce the likelihood of a heart attack or artery damage by eating lots of fresh fruits and vegetables. Meats, and more specifically red meats such as pork and beef, contribute to the buildup of plaque in the arteries, which impacts the function of the heart. Over time, this narrows the arteries and reduces blood flow, which increases blood pressure and the risk of a heart attack.

- Vegan foods reduce inflammation caused by animal-based foods, which are highly acidic. Chronic conditions such as arthritis can cause the body to swell from inflammation, which can result in pain in specific areas of the body, and this can spread and worsen over time. While inflammation is the body's response to fighting infection and disease, it can occur incorrectly and over long time periods, thus causing constant pain. When it becomes chronic, pain management is often prescribed in the form of medication and modifications to the diet. Plant-based foods provide relief by reducing and even preventing or stopping inflammation completely once veganism becomes a regular part of your diet.

- There is a reduced risk of developing type 2 diabetes when switching from an animal-based or lacto-ovo vegetarian diet. In fact, some research indicates that the risk of developing diabetes is reduced by half. If you've already been diagnosed with diabetes, adopting a vegan diet is a much better option to manage your sugar levels. This is because the all-natural sources of sugar in fruits and vegetables are unprocessed and not excessive. When eating an animal-based diet, there is less attention to natural food sources in many cases, as vegetables and other foods take a second or third level of importance in many meals which place meat as the featured item. When you switch to plant-based eating, the quality of your food becomes more important because it's absorbed quickly, as the body digests it more efficiently than animal-based foods.

- Studies have shown a decreased risk of cancer in people who follow a plant-based diet and avoid animal and dairy products. This research indicates a link between eating red meat and cancer, due to the amount of trans fats and carcinogens these meats often contain. One of the most specific cancers that are prevented by eating a vegan diet is colon cancer. Carcinogens contribute to the accumulation of abnormal cell growth, forming cancer. In fact, proteins found in meat can increase the growth of cancerous cells and speed up the process, while vegan or vegetable-based proteins do not have the same effect.

- Eating vegan foods is better for digestion and promotes regularity while preventing constipation. This is also a great way to increase your metabolic rate and works well with a regular exercise routine. It's virtually impossible to become obese or significantly overweight while following a plant-based diet.

- You'll generally feel better and any bloating or gastric issues, including cramps, will usually disappear. A vegan diet is excellent for women of all ages and can alleviate the symptoms of menstrual cramps and discomfort as well as the side effects associated with entering menopause. A plant-based diet has all the ingredients needed to improve your way of life, including your mental, physical, and psychological well being.

Aside from the general benefits of a vegan diet, there are plenty of reasons why more athletes are going plant-based. It's become a much easier way to live and eat, with all the new meat and dairy alternatives and overall popularity. These reasons are research-based and the effects, when experienced, provide many advantages for an active lifestyle, which are explored in the next section below. (The Health

9

Benefits of Eating a Plant-based diet and How to Get Started, n.d.)

How Can Athletes Benefit From a Vegan Diet?

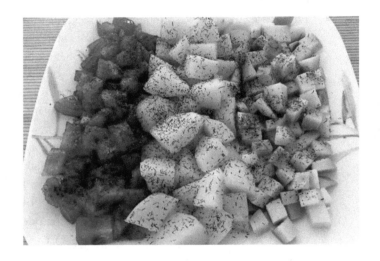

The benefits of a vegan diet are plentiful for bodybuilders, marathon participants, and all other types of athletes. Contrary to the myths and misconceptions about plant-based eating, there are many sources of protein, calcium, vitamins, and other nutrients to support the healthy development of muscle and tissue growth at a cellular level. A vegan diet is primarily based on natural, whole foods, leaving little or no room for processed products. It's also simpler to prepare and plan vegan meals while enjoying the advantages of creating new, delicious recipes and finding a wide range of options beyond dairy and meat.

What are the specific benefits of ditching animal products for plant-based eating? First and foremost, if you live and thrive in a physically active lifestyle, you'll need to increase your caloric intake. As an athlete, your BMI or bodyweight will be within a healthy range, and cutting calories is not recommended. At the same time, it's important not to consume an excessive number of calories, which is where a vegan diet provides some essential balance. By sticking with plant-based foods, you'll get all the nutrients and get the right amount of calories you need to maintain and improve your body and athletic performance.

An athletic lifestyle is a healthy way to live, though your risk of heart disease can remain the same if you continue eating an animal-based diet. In fact, bodybuilding and other strength training exercises can increase your heart's size and require it to function more and harder, which can be dangerous, especially if you eat a high amount of red meat and trans fats found in processed foods. A plant-based diet reduces this risk by close to 40 percent, which is significant and can help you avoid the potential for cardiac arrest in the future. You'll also have healthier arteries, blood flow, and nutrient absorption, which is due to your blood becoming more viscous or thick. When this occurs, your blood is able to transport nutrients more effectively throughout the body. This also keeps your cholesterol levels in check by preventing them from getting too high, which can contribute to many other health issues. As nutrients are better transported within the body, you will have a greater supply of oxygen which feeds the muscles and improves performance.

With a diet high in fresh fruits and vegetables, people who eat vegan will consume more antioxidants than their meat-based diet counterparts. For this reason, they are better equipped to fight and prevent diseases caused by the production of free radicals in the body. Free radicals are produced when processed, toxic foods are consumed. They can harm and interfere with the body's natural functions by encouraging the growth of tumors, cancerous cells, and various infections. Antioxidants, on the other hand, fight against and prevent the development of free radicals, protecting the body from them. When you increase the amount of these nutrients in your diet, you'll enjoy a greatly reduced risk of developing these conditions. Berries, citrus fruits, dark leafy greens, and pomegranates are great sources of antioxidants. Chia seeds are another excellent source and can be added to smoothies and plant-based desserts easily.

As you become familiar with all the options within a plant-based diet, along with these and other benefits, you'll find there are many useful options for vegan foods, including unlimited recipes and ideas, all of which are delicious and easy to prepare.

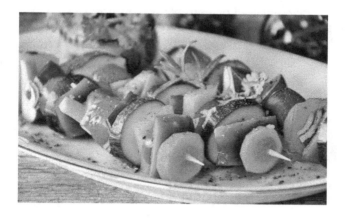

Before you dive into the world of plant-based eating, here are some important steps and suggestions to keep you focused and successful once you begin:

1. It's important to adapt to a plant-based diet on your own terms and at your own pace. Not everyone can ditch all animal products in one day and switch completely to vegan without making changes in stages over several weeks, even months. Every individual is different, and once you discover what works best for you, you'll be able to make those changes within your own time frame. For example, you may start by cutting down on meat or starting with dairy first. Cut out the animal foods that you don't eat as often, or eliminate one specific item at

a time such as beef, chicken, or certain milk products.

2. Swap meat and dairy-based foods for a close vegan alternative. For example, if you normally enjoy a ham sandwich or tuna salad wrap, you may want to try hummus and smoked tempeh or tofu with sprouts as a tasty way to move into your vegan options. There are also vegan cheese slices that have similar flavors to their dairy counterparts, which can be used in the same way on subs, wraps, and sandwiches. A grilled portobello mushroom works well in place of a meat burger, and lentil stew instead of beef soup. Hummus and eggplant dips and spreads work as excellent replacements for mayonnaise and cheese options.

3. Don't be afraid to try new foods, including fruits and vegetables you may usually choose on your regular grocery trips. Shop at local food markets and stores specializing in imported goods. Try at least one new fruit or vegetable every two weeks, including something you might not usually eat. For some people, this might be eggplant, squash, or kale. Some of these options may not seem as favorable until you use them in a recipe. You'll discover a new exciting way to use plant-based foods. Squash, for example, may seem unappetizing to some because they haven't experienced the mellow aroma of butternut squash soup or as a roasted vegetable. If you don't feel initially comfortable trying a new food on your own, find a restaurant with the specific item in a dish. Buffets or vegan eateries are a good start and

can offer many new ideas and flavors to try, inspiring and expanding your palate.

4. Get familiar with all the plant-based foods that provide essential nutrients, and make them a part of your regular shopping list. Beans, grains, greens, apples, berries, avocados, soy food, and other vegan options are a great foundation to build from. Consider your proteins, minerals (iron, copper, magnesium, etc.), vitamins, fiber, and other nutrients by organizing them into a chart or categories and listing foods that contain a significant source of each, as follows:

    a. Protein - beans, soy (tofu, tempeh, miso),

    b. Potassium - bananas, watermelon, potatoes

    c. Vitamin C - oranges, lemon, lime, grapefruit, peppers, apples

    d. Vitamin B/beta carotene - carrots, squash, yams/sweet potatoes

    e. Antioxidants - berries, chia seeds

    f. Healthy fats - avocado, flax seeds, hemp seeds, coconut oil, MCT oil

    g. Iron - leafy greens, cabbage, beetroot

5. Do you have allergies or food sensitivities? Many people discover these early in life, and sometimes, intolerance for certain foods develop later in life. Peanuts, seafood, shellfish, and gluten items are common foods that certain people become allergic to or must avoid, either due to mild reactions or fatal consequences in some rare circumstances. Take note of any sensitivities you have and notice whether or not they are vegan. Many intolerances

are dairy-related because some people experience difficulty with digesting lactose, which is a sugar contained in milk. Fortunately, you won't need to worry about animal-based foods that cause reactions. Going vegan most likely means reducing the number of foods you must avoid while allowing you to try new options.

6. Think about the plant-based foods you currently enjoy and make them a part of your diet right away. This includes meals you eat at restaurants, buffet options, and snacks you may enjoy on the go when you're commuting to work or school. Hot cereal, granola, bananas, hummus and crackers, guacamole, and vegetable side dishes are examples of what you may enjoy already and may continue to include in your diet when you completely switch to vegan foods.

7. Try adapting some of your favorite meat or dairy-based foods into vegan versions, such as a vegetable pasta sauce instead of meat sauce, or curried tofu instead of chicken. You may find referencing a recipe and substituting specific items with vegan options works best, or if you are a more experienced cook, try your own creations based on the dishes that inspire you.

8. Some people are comfortable with lacto ovo vegetarianism, which can be a step towards veganism. The lacto ovo method of eating includes dairy and eggs, without meat. For other people, a pescatarian diet works well by allowing them to eat fish while cutting out all other meats. Both of these

forms of semi-vegetarianism are paths towards a fully plant-based diet.

Take time out of your schedule to explore vegan menu items, new vegan restaurants (these are usually more common than you'd think, especially in urban areas), and grocery items. While some vegan versions of cheese, dairy, and meat may seem unappealing at first, you may be pleasantly surprised by the variety of options that are available. The days of unappetizing, bland vegan substitutes are far gone, and a variety of flavorful, spicy, and aromatic blends of vegan cheese (soy or vegetable-based), coconut-cultured yogurts, nut-based and soy milk options awaits. Soy-based meat substitutes have greatly improved to the point of being indistinguishable from actual meat products, such as hamburgers and hot dogs.

Beans, legumes, and grains are an excellent and nutritious way to enhance your meals and build a foundation for them. Rice is one of the most versatile foods and can provide much-needed energy in the form of carbohydrates before a major tournament or marathon. Lentils, kidney beans, black beans, and chickpeas are all great sources of both protein and fiber. Use as many options as possible, including quinoa, couscous, oats, barley, and many other grains, as they will boost the nutrient and energy value of every meal. Explore veganism in your own way, and take your time so that you become familiar and comfortable with the switch from meat-based to plant-based. (Cook Creatively, 2016)

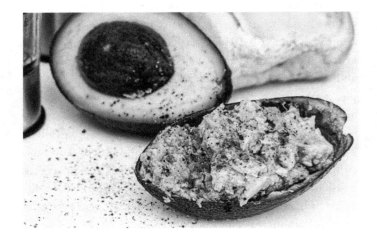

To maximize the benefits of a plant-based diet, there are some practices to keep in mind. These actions can increase the benefits of what vegan eating can do for your body and overall health:

- Eat raw whenever possible. Enjoying a meal with sauteed and stir-fried vegetables can be excellent, but if you can, try to increase the number of meals with raw food options, such as salads, hummus with a handful of peppers, cucumbers, carrots, and celery, or a fruit salad. Take advantage of raw produce toppings on veggie burgers or portobello mushroom patties. Enjoy an orange or apple in

18

between meals as a snack or a pomegranate with your morning cereal.

- Add healthy fats to your diet. This includes monounsaturated and polyunsaturated fats, which help boost your cognitive function and provide many nutrients. You can find these in avocados, coconut oil, olive oil, nuts, and seeds. Incorporating a small handful of nuts and seeds or an avocado each day will ensure you get the right amount of fats you need in your diet. Flax and hemp seeds are also good options.

- To reduce sugar in your diet, use fruit as part of or all of a dessert option. For example, a raw, sliced mango with coconut cream is a tasty option, or try lightly baked apples sprinkled with cinnamon. A bowl of fresh berries in almond milk with or without cereal can be an excellent option for breakfast or a midday snack. If you're often on the go, bananas and apples are great options as well.

- Try a new food item once every week or two weeks. This might be something you've never tasted before, like a rare exotic fruit or vegetable, or a seed or nuts that are not commonly found in regular grocery stores. Make a point of visiting and shopping at foreign food markets and ask questions about trying new foods. Jackfruit, papaya, guava, and taro are examples of foods that are emerging in popularity in vegan cuisine and recipes.

- Add a handful of nuts and seeds to your diet whenever you need a quick snack. Making a habit of having a healthy source of eating available will make it easier.

Chapter 2: Vegan Recipes for Athletes Before the Workout

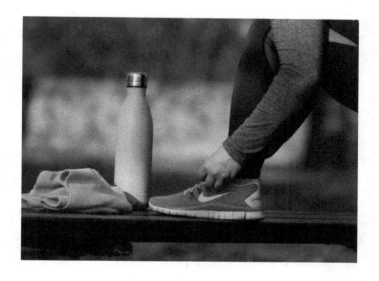

Before you head for the gym or embark on a bicycle ride, you'll want to add a quality source of fuel to provide enough energy for building muscle, tissue, and endurance. The types of food you choose may depend on the type of exercise and your goals. If your aim is to lose weight and slim down, choose high energy options with low carbohydrates and calories. Fiber is an excellent nutrient to have in every meal. Protein is also vital, though you don't need to eat large amounts at each meal to gain the most benefit. In fact, North Americans tend to eat excessive amounts of protein in a traditional meat-based diet, which isn't fully digested and used by our bodies. A vegan diet provides just the right amount for our body to use for building muscle tissue. Many other nutrients are included in the meals below, such as vitamins, antioxidants, and minerals.

Smoothies

Avocado Coconut Smoothie

A good source of healthy fats and fiber, avocados provide an excellent source of energy to burn before the workout. They also satisfy your hunger for a while, as they are filling as a snack and more effective in a smoothie. Paired with coconut milk, avocados are blended into a thick milkshake along with a natural sweetener. For additional fiber and a dose of potassium, add one banana to this drink as well.

- 1 avocado (ripe)
- 1 ½ cups of coconut milk
- 2 teaspoons of natural or low carb sweetener
- Dash of vanilla (optional)
- 1 banana (optional)

Place all ingredients into the blender, starting with the avocado and coconut milk, to mix. Add in the sweetener, vanilla, and banana. Continue to blend and monitor the thickness, adding a bit of extra coconut milk as needed, then serve. For a boost of protein, add one tablespoon of vanilla powder (hemp or soy-based protein) during the blend.

Mango Cardamom Pistachio Smoothie

This smoothie can be prepared with the option of adding coconut cultured yogurt or almond milk (or another non-dairy milk). Mangoes are naturally sweet in flavor and thicken well in recipes and smoothies, which makes them easy to work with.

- 1 large or 2 small mangoes
- 2 cups of almond or coconut milk
- 2 teaspoons of natural or low carb sweetener
- 1 teaspoon of cardamom
- 2 tablespoons of crushed pistachios
- ¼ teaspoon of vanilla

When choosing mangoes for this recipe, ensure they are soft and very ripe so that they are effortless to peel, pit, and slice. Add the mangoes, coconut milk, pistachios, sweetener, vanilla, and cardamom to the blender and pulse until smooth, then serve.

Banana and Berries Smoothie

This smoothie is prepared with a banana, which is an excellent source of energy, providing up to one hour prior to a workout. Bananas, like avocado, are a good thickening agent for smoothies and milkshakes. Berries are full of antioxidants, fiber, and vitamin C, which are important for your daily requirements.

- 1 cup of fresh or frozen berries (cherries, strawberries, raspberries, blueberries, blackberries, or any combination of these)
- 1 ripe banana
- 2 cups of almond or coconut milk
- 1 teaspoon of maple syrup or low carb sweetener

Add all items into the blender and pulse until smooth, which usually takes about 45 seconds, then serve.

Cocoa Peanut Butter Smoothie

If you have a chocolate craving, you don't have to wait until dessert. Natural cocoa or vegan dark chocolate can be easily added to your smoothie along with a good dose of protein in the form of peanut butter. Almond, hazelnut, or other nut butters can be used instead, if available. Nut butters are also an excellent source of healthy fats and provide a lot of energy before a workout or as a complete breakfast.

- ¾ cups of peanut butter (smooth)
- 1-2 teaspoons of raw sugar, maple syrup, or low carb sweetener
- 2 cups of almond or soy milk (unsweetened, unflavored)
- 3-4 tablespoons of cocoa or dark vegan chocolate (melted or in powder form)

Add all items in a blender and pulse for 45 seconds, until smooth, then serve.

Tahini Coconut Smoothie

The tahini coconut smoothie is ideal with or without fruit. Adding one banana is an option and compliments the smooth taste of tahini, which combines well with coconut or almond milk. Shredded or fresh coconut is another choice you can add along with the coconut milk.

- 2 cups of coconut milk
- 2 teaspoons of shredded or fresh coconut
- 1 cup of tahini
- 2 teaspoons of maple syrup
- 1 tablespoon of vegan protein (soy, hemp, or nut-based are all good options)
- 1 banana (optional)

Mix the coconut milk and tahini in the blender, until smooth, then add in the remaining ingredients before mixing for 30 seconds longer, and serve.

Pumpkin Protein Smoothie

Canned or fresh (seasonal) pumpkin is great for creating a smoothie and may be combined with traditional pumpkin spice, a combination of nutmeg, cinnamon, and cloves, along with either coconut or almond milk. While pumpkins contain their own source of protein, this smoothie boosts the amount by adding a heaping tablespoon of either pumpkin protein, hemp, or soy protein powder. If you have yet to become familiar with these options, try purchasing them in a bulk store in small amounts.

- 1 cup of pureed pumpkin
- 1 ½ cups of almond or coconut milk
- 1 teaspoon of vanilla extract
- 2 teaspoons of maple syrup or natural sweetener (low carb)
- 1 teaspoon of nutmeg
- 1 teaspoon of cinnamon
- ¼ teaspoon of cloves

Combine all the ingredients into a bowl first, mash the pumpkin flesh with the spices, then add the almond or coconut milk. Pour the mixture into a blender, add the sweetener and vanilla, and pulse until smooth, then serve. For a twist on the flavor, add one banana and an extra ½ cup of non-dairy milk.

Peanut Butter and Jelly Smoothie

You can skip the sandwich and try this fun peanut butter based smoothie with a topping of natural berry jelly, jam, or marmalade. When choosing a marmalade, unless you create your own homemade jam, use the most natural, low sugar option with no artificial ingredients. The smoothie base is relatively simple, consisting of just a few ingredients:

- ½ cup of peanut butter (smooth)
- 1 ½ cups of oat, almond, or soy milk
- 1 teaspoon of sweetener

- 1 banana (optional)

Combine all the above ingredients in a blender and pulse for 35-40 seconds, then serve and top with a dollop of one of the following:

- Orange marmalade
- Strawberry, blueberry, or raspberry jelly or jam

Adding fresh berries on top, or blending with the ingredients, is another great option for this recipe.

Almond Date Smoothie

Combining high fiber content with healthy fats and protein can be done with just a few ingredients. Almonds contain both fiber and healthy fats, which are boosted with the addition of fiber-rich dates. If dates are unavailable, prunes are another option.

- 2 cups of almond or coconut milk
- ½ cup crushed almonds
- ½ cup of pitted, packed dates
- 1 tablespoon coconut cream
- 1 teaspoon almond extract

Add all the ingredients into a blender and pulse until smooth. It may help to blend or crush the dates first, separately, so they mix easier with the remaining ingredients. Serve on ice, or add ice to crush when blending the smoothie.

Pineapple Coconut Mango Smoothie

This smoothie is the perfect tropical fruit mix, providing a decent boost of fiber and vitamins in one serving. Papayas, peaches, and guavas are also great options to substitute or add along with the other fruits. Coconut milk adds some healthy fats and a mild flavor to balance out the fruit medley.

- 1 cup of raw or frozen pineapple, chopped
- ½ cup of frozen or raw mango, sliced
- 2 cups of coconut milk
- 1 teaspoon of coconut oil
- 1 teaspoon of vanilla extract
- 2 teaspoons of maple syrup or low carb sweetener

Combine all the ingredients into a blender, and pulse for 30-40 seconds. Serve and top with shredded coconut. If all fruits used in the recipe are fresh, you may choose to crush ice and add it to the smoothie to chill.

Kefir Coconut Smoothie

This smoothie is made with coconut-based kefir, a non-dairy version of this fermented drink, and coconut milk. A dash of sweetener and coconut oil is added for more vitamins and healthy fats.

- 2 cups of coconut milk
- 1 cup of kefir (plain, unsweetened)

- 2 tablespoons of maple syrup or low carb sweetener
- 1 teaspoon of coconut oil
- 1 banana

Add the kefir, coconut oil, and coconut milk to the blender and pulse for 30-40 seconds. Pour in the sweetener and the banana, then blend again, and serve.

Energy Bars

Energy bars, also known as protein bars, are an excellent snack and quick way to gain a powerful dose of energy in a short timeframe. This is especially important if you find yourself skipping a meal or delaying dinner due to a busy schedule. For this reason, it's important to ensure that you're getting the most out of your energy bar by packing it with loads of nutrients specifically designed for your workout goals. Many store-bought brands are high in sugar and preservatives, despite claiming to be natural and without any artificial ingredients.

Creating your own energy bar is rewarding and satisfying; you will know what it contains, and this will alleviate any concerns about the quality you are getting. Energy bars are often protein-based, and there are many vegan sources of protein to include and consider: hemp, soy, almond (nut-based powders and protein), pumpkin, and many others. To prepare ahead of time, you may want to visit a local bulk or natural food store to determine the variety of plant-based protein options they offer. Then you can budget and plan ahead accordingly.

Peanut Butter and Oat Energy Bars

Peanut and other nut-based butters are ideal for creating energy bars, including this simple recipe. Oats are added to create a healthy, balanced source of energy, with a wealth of nutrients and fuel for your workout. It's best to consume a half hour or more before your workout, to ensure you digest the nutrients well before starting your activity. This recipe contains only three ingredients, and these are easily blended without any baking.

- ¾ cups of peanut butter
- 1 cup of dates (pitted)
- ½ cup of oats (regular or gluten-free)

Combine all three ingredients into a food processor and pulse until smooth. If the ingredients don't mix easily, try blending a portion of the dates and oats with the full amount of peanut butter, until they are well blended. Then add in the rest of the dates and oats and continue blending until the batter is ready. Pour batter into a 3-inch high resealable container or baking tray and press down firmly and evenly. Place the container in the freezer for a minimum of two hours, then transfer to the refrigerator. Serve from the refrigerator, and be cautious not to store at room temperature or the bars may soften and stick. These bars keep well chilled for up to two weeks.

Maple Almond Energy Bars

This is a tasty recipe that incorporates almonds rich in protein and healthy fats with maple syrup. Only a small portion is needed to provide a significant boost before heading to the gym. The maple syrup can be replaced with a low carb maple-flavored sweetener if you follow a low carb diet. If maple syrup is used, make sure it is the natural option and not an artificially flavored, high fructose corn syrup variety. Agave can also be substituted where maple syrup is not available.

- 1 cup of packed dates, pitted
- ½ cup of almond butter
- 3 tablespoons of maple syrup
- 1 cup of roasted almonds
- 1 ¼ cups of rolled oats

Roasted almonds can be store-bought or raw almonds can be roasted at home in the oven. To create the homemade version, lightly coat the raw almonds with grapeseed oil and place evenly on a baking tray. Bake for 5-6 minutes in a preheated oven at 350 degrees. This can be done without oil as well, which is known as dry roasting. When this process is done, remove from the oven and set aside to cool for 10-15 minutes.

To prepare the bars, pulse the dates in a food processor until they are smooth, then remove and combine with almonds and oats in a large bowl. In a small saucepan, heat the almond butter and maple syrup on low, and stir to combine both ingredients thoroughly. Pour mixture over the oats, almonds, and dates, and fold together evenly. Transfer to a baking tray or casserole dish and firmly press down the mixture so that it coats the bottom of the tray. Refrigerate for two hours minimum, then serve. For best results, place in the freezer for two hours, then transfer to the refrigerator to store until serving. Slice the bars into 8-10 portions to serve.

Tahini and Chocolate Energy Bars

Tahini is a protein-rich butter that works just as well in most recipes which typically use peanut and almond butter as ingredients. It's often found in grocery or specialty stores, and it's used as one of the ingredients in creating hummus. If you prefer the homemade option, you can blend ¼ cup of sesame seeds in a food processor or blender with a small amount of olive oil, until smooth, then refrigerate or store in a sealable container at room temperature, unless you're ready to use it right away.

- 2 cups of dates, pitted and packed
- ¾ cups of hemp seeds
- ½ cup of tahini
- Dash of sea salt
- 3 tablespoons of almond milk
- ½ cup of chocolate protein powder (soy or another vegan-based protein option)
- 4 tablespoons of cocoa powder

To create the dough, add all the ingredients to a food processor and blend until smooth. This may take several attempts, if they do not initially mix well, and can be done in batches to achieve the desired effect. The entire mix should form a dough that is easy to spread. Line a tray with parchment paper and transfer the dough to the center, pressing it down and evenly to coat the entire surface. Cover with plastic wrap and place in the freezer for four hours, then slice into 12-14 portions and serve. Keep the remaining bars in the refrigerator.

Cashew Energy Bars

Cashews are another great source of both protein and fiber and make an excellent option for creating energy bars. Cashew butter can often be found in natural food stores, and a growing number of supermarkets now offer it as well. Like peanut butter energy bars, these are created with minimal ingredients.

- 1 cup of dates, pitted and packed
- ½ cup of cashew butter
- ½ cup of oats
- 1 tablespoon of chia seeds
- 2 tablespoons of maple syrup

Mix all the ingredients in the food processor. Pulse in batches, starting with cashew butter and maple syrup, then gradually add in other ingredients and continue to blend. Once completed, transfer the mixture to a baking tray and press evenly. Place in the freezer for four hours, then move into the refrigerator to store. Bars can be sliced and served, and they should be stored in the refrigerator until used.

Hemp Protein Energy Bars

Hemp protein is an excellent source of energy and can be easily added to any energy bar recipe. Healthy fats are another advantage to hemp seeds and protein and can be added to cereals, smoothies, and salads. These bars are simple and easy to create, without the need for an oven or stovetop cooking.

- 2 teaspoons of hemp protein
- 1 cup of nut-based butter (almond, peanut, hazelnut, or cashew butter, or any combination of these options)
- 2 teaspoons of low carb sweetener or maple syrup
- ½ cup of oats
- 1 teaspoon of chia seeds
- 1 teaspoon of cinnamon

In a small or medium bowl, mash your choice of nut-based butter with the hemp protein, then combine the remaining ingredients, mixing thoroughly until a batter is formed. Transfer the batter to a lined baking tray with parchment paper, pressing down firmly, then place in the freezer for at least three hours. Transfer to the refrigerator, slice, and serve. Bars can remain sealed in the refrigerator for up to one week.

Snacks

Kale Chips

Kale chips are easy and quick to prepare with just three main ingredients and a regular oven. Kale is an ideal vegetable for chips due to its high level of iron, calcium, protein, and fiber. The texture of kale varies depending on the type, which ranges from flat to curly, and either green, red, or black in color. Any variety can be used for kale chips.

- 1 bunch of kale (any variety)
- 2 tablespoons of olive oil or coconut oil
- 2-3 teaspoons of sea salt

Prepare the kale by washing and thoroughly drying each leaf, then removing the stems and slicing each leaf into one or two-inch pieces. Lightly coat each piece in olive oil and place on a baking tray (this works best on a tray prepared with parchment paper), then sprinkle with sea salt, coating each slice evenly. Bake at 350 degrees for 8-10 minutes, then serve. Keep an eye on the oven, as the kale is usually ready within this time frame. The chips should be dry and crispy, not wet or burnt.

Other options to consider include coating the chips with cumin, cayenne, or chili pepper.

Hummus and Vegetables

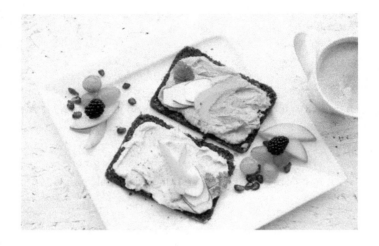

Hummus is a tasty, protein-rich dip that can accompany biscuits and vegetables or can be used as a spread on a wrap or sandwich. Traditionally, hummus is created with chickpeas or a similar legume, with tahini (also known as sesame butter), lemon, garlic, cumin, and olive oil. Spices and additional flavors can be added to enhance the taste of this dip, such as chili powder or curry, or it can be blended with vegetables such as beetroot and avocado. What is one of the best reasons to incorporate hummus into your plant-based diet? It's a favorite dish among vegans and non-vegans equally. This dip can be a great way to bridge the change from dairy-based spreads, such as mayonnaise and cream cheese, when enjoying sandwiches and vegetables.

- 1 can of chickpeas (drained and rinsed)
- ½ cup of tahini (sesame butter)
- 2 tablespoons of olive oil
- 1 teaspoon of cumin
- 2 teaspoons of lemon juice (freshly squeezed)
- ½ teaspoon of sea salt
- 2-3 crushed cloves of garlic
- Dash of black pepper

Combine the drained and rinsed chickpeas in a blender and add in the tahini, olive oil, lemon juice, and garlic. Pulse for roughly 60 seconds, then add the remaining ingredients and continue to blend. Taste test the dip to ensure it is flavored as desired, and add more lemon, tahini, garlic, or other ingredients. Then serve as a dip or spread. Cucumbers, carrots, celery make a great companion to hummus on a platter or as a snack.

Avocado Toast

If you need a quick way to fuel up before a workout, the combination of toast and avocado works well, as this combination provides an excellent source of carbohydrates, fiber, and healthy fats. Rye or whole grain bread is recommended for this snack. The avocado should be ripe, though not too mushy, so that it can be sliced gently for each slice of bread. This sandwich is best served open-faced.

- 1 avocado
- 1 teaspoon of vegan butter

- 2 slices of rye bread
- 1 teaspoon of sesame seeds

Toast both slices of bread, then butter each and place on a plate. Slice the ripe avocado, after removing the shell and pit, then assemble evenly on each piece of bread. Sprinkle with sesame seeds, then serve.

Baked Onion Rings

If you enjoy the savory taste of onions, either baked or sauteed, you'll enjoy these health-conscious onion rings easily assembled and made in the oven within minutes. Large, red onions work best for this recipe, though white or yellow onions are another option. Slice large rings and separate them to prepare ahead of time. Rinse each of the rings and onions under cold water to prevent or reduce their effects on your eyes when preparing them. Red onions are slightly less pungent, and sweeter, which creates a unique flavor for this snack. Onions provide a great source of vitamin C and fiber, while almond flour and milk add some protein and healthy fat.

- 1 cup of almond flour
- 2 large red onions, sliced into rings
- 2 tablespoons of olive oil
- 2-3 teaspoons of almond milk (unsweetened, unflavored)
- 1 teaspoon of Cajun spice
- 1 teaspoon of black pepper

- ½ teaspoon of sea salt

In a small bowl, add the almond milk, olive oil, and sea salt, stirring for a few seconds. Add the almond flour, Cajun spice, and black pepper to a second bowl, and mix with a fork. Slice each of the onions, run them under cold water, then pat them dry. Separate each group of rings sliced from the onions separately. Prepare a baking tray by lining with parchment paper. Dip each onion ring first in the almond milk-sea salt mix, coating evenly, then dip into the bowl of almond flour, Cajun spice, and black pepper. Ensure each ring is covered completely, and evenly, before placing on the tray. Bake in a preheated oven at 350 degrees for approximately 10-11 minutes on each side, until lightly browned and crispy. Remove, and serve with coconut-cultured plain yogurt or vegan sour cream.

Chia Seed Pudding

This is an easy recipe to prepare and is often best to create the night before, allowing the chia seeds to absorb the other ingredients and flavors. Chia seeds are considered a superfood, due to the high density and variety of nutrients they contain: fiber, protein, calcium, antioxidants, and vitamins. Just a small amount of chia seeds can go a long way to improve your health and boost the quality of your diet

- ½ cup of chia seeds
- ¼ cup of coconut cream

- 1 cup of coconut milk
- 2 tablespoons of maple syrup (or low carb sweetener)
- 1 teaspoon of vanilla extract

Combine all the above ingredients in a medium bowl and whisk together. You may notice the chia seeds stick together, which is natural, though most of them will combine with the coconut milk and cream. Taste test to ensure you don't need to add more sweetener, then transfer to a resealable container and refrigerate for at least two hours. If refrigerating overnight, chia seed pudding can be served in the morning for breakfast, either before work or the gym. The following toppings may also be considered:

- Crushed pistachio nuts, peanuts, sliced almonds, walnuts and/or pecans
- Fresh berries, sliced peaches, mangoes and/or apples
- Shredded coconut or flakes
- A dusting of cinnamon or cardamom, to create a rice pudding-like taste
- A light sprinkling of brown or raw sugar
- Pumpkin or sesame seeds

Experiment with a variety of toppings, flavors, and ingredients. Toppings can also be added before, as ingredients, when mixing the chia seeds with the milk and cream. For a better blend, add your choice of fruit with the coconut or almond milk and pulse in a food processor, before combining with the remaining ingredients to create the pudding.

Pear and Apple Compote

Pears and apples make excellent snacks on their own, especially when you have little or no time to prepare a light meal in advance. They also combine to create a tasty compote, which can be used as a topping on crepes or green salads, or simply enjoyed as a dessert on its own or a snack.

- 2 large apples, any variety, peeled, cored, and sliced
- 1 large pear, peeled, cored, and sliced (or 2 small pears)
- 1 inch of fresh ginger root
- ¼ slice of lemon peel
- 1 tablespoon of apple cider vinegar
- 2 cinnamon sticks, or 1 tablespoon of ground cinnamon
- 2 tablespoons of raw sugar or low carb sweetener
- 3 tablespoons of maple syrup

To prepare the compote, combine the apples, pears (both sliced in small half-inch or one-inch pieces), ginger root, lemon peel, apple cider vinegar, sweetener or raw sugar and cinnamon sticks into a large or medium-sized cooking pot. Cook on medium until ingredients are brought to a simmer, and pour in a small amount of water (2-3 tablespoons) or the equivalent amount in vinegar, and continue to stew. Continue to stew the ingredients until the pears and apples are tender, then remove from the stove to serve. Add as a topping to vegan ice cream and drizzle maple syrup on top.

Roasted Squash Seeds

Pumpkin seeds are popular as a roasted snack, though seeds from any variety of squash can also be used for the same recipe. They are not only nutritious but tasty and prepared in much the same way as oven-roasted pumpkin seeds. If you have a leftover squash from a recipe, always remove, rinse and dry the seeds, then refrigerate them for up to one or two days before preparing them for roasting. This can be done easily with just three ingredients and a few minutes in the oven.

- 1 cup of raw squash seeds (make sure they are rinsed and dried, with no squash flesh attached to them)
- 2 tablespoons of olive oil
- 1 teaspoon of sea salt

Prepare a large or medium baking sheet with parchment paper. Lightly coat each of the seeds, and place them evenly spaced apart on the tray. Sprinkle lightly with sea salt, and if desired, add black pepper or other spices, such as cumin, chili pepper and/or Cajun spice for a flavor twist. Bake in the oven for 18-22 minutes, until toasted and crispy, but not burnt. Keep an eye on the oven after 15 minutes to avoid burning any of the seeds. Once they are done, remove from the oven and place in a bowl or plate to cool slightly, then serve. Seeds will last in an airtight container for up to one week in the pantry, or up to two weeks in the refrigerator.

Cinnamon Roasted Pumpkin Seeds

Pumpkin seeds are a popular snack and are often enjoyed roasted with sea salt. This recipe provides a twist on the common salted variety by adding cinnamon and sweetener or raw sugar instead. This is an ideal way to satisfy a sweet tooth craving without excessive sugar and additives. Raw pumpkin seeds are best fresh and can be collected from the inside of the pumpkin after carving and separating them from the flesh.

- 1 cup of raw pumpkin seeds
- 2 teaspoons of cinnamon (ground)
- 1 teaspoon of raw sugar or granulated low carb sugar
- 3 tablespoons of coconut oil, melted at room temperature

Clean all the seeds, removing the flesh and washing them, then pat dry. Prepare a baking sheet with parchment paper and lightly coat each of the seeds in coconut oil. Place them on the tray, ensuring they are evenly spaced. Gently mix the sugar or low carb sugar with the cinnamon and sprinkle lightly over the seeds. Bake in a preheated oven at 350 degrees for 16-18 minutes, or until seeds are crispy and toasty but not burnt. For best results, start with a small batch to gauge the accurate time frame for baking and prevent burning when preparing a large batch. Remove from the oven to cool, then serve. Toasted seeds can be kept at room temperature in a sealed container for up to two weeks.

Chapter 3: Vegan Recipes for Athletes After the Workout

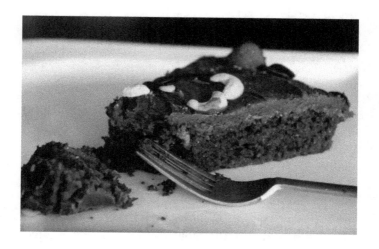

After the workout, you'll need a nourishing meal to replenish your body and nutrient levels. Each of these recipes is simple, easy to prepare, and provides a tasty experience. Every meal is high in vitamins, minerals, and other nutrients to boost your overall health.

Soups and Broths

Enjoying a soup or broth is an ideal way to get the most out of a basic meal. It's a great way to replenish your body's energy, without overeating or feeling too full. Vegetables, mushrooms, and miso soup bases are commonly used in a vegan diet. They can be found conveniently in most grocery stores or created from scratch using leftover vegetable peelings and shavings.

Miso Soup (Basic Recipe)

If miso soup is familiar to you, it might be due to its popularity in sushi restaurants and as a base for soups and sauces in Asian cuisine. It's a nutrient-dense form of fermented soy, which contains B12, calcium, protein, and vitamins that provide the building blocks for a healthy body. Miso is often available in paste form, requiring just one or two teaspoons mixed with boiling water for a simple cup or bowl of soup. There are three types of miso: white, yellow, and red. White and yellow varieties are often used as a soup base, due to having a mild to moderate flavor, whereas red miso is more commonly used in sauces and dips.

- 2 cups of water
- 1 teaspoon of miso paste
- 1 green onion
- ¼ cup of sliced tofu
- 1 sheet of seaweed (nori)

To prepare the soup, bring two cups of water to a boil, and stir in the miso paste. Continue to stir until the paste is dissolved, and reduce the heat to low. Slice the tofu into small, ½-inch cubes, and chop the green onion and seaweed

46

into small pieces. Add these ingredients into the soup, stirring and continue to stew for several minutes, then serve.

Ramen Soup

Ramen noodles are either known as the inexpensive option for a budget grocery list or as a dish that is quickly gaining in popularity in Japanese restaurants, alongside sushi and teriyaki dishes. Ramen soup bowls can include any variety of vegetables and spices, according to your taste. For maximum nutrient value, it's best to add dark green vegetables, along with sprouts and other fresh vegetables.

To prepare this dish, a larger portion of miso soup is prepared and may be combined with vegetable broth, either store-bought or homemade.

- 4 cups of water
- 2 tablespoons of miso paste
- 1 cup of tofu, cut into cubes
- 1 cup of sliced broccoli
- 1 small onion, diced
- 1 carrot, diced
- 1 cup of sprouts
- 1 teaspoon of black pepper
- 1 handful of ramen or rice noodles
- 1 teaspoon of crushed chilies

Boil four cups of water on the stovetop and add the miso paste, gradually stirring until dissolved. Break in half, and add the ramen noodles and continue cooking on high until they are soft. Add the chilies, small onion, tofu, and black pepper, then continue to stir. Combine and add the remaining ingredients and stew on medium-low, until tender, and serve.

Butternut Squash Soup

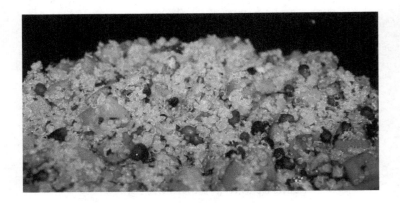

Squash is a tasty, mellow-flavored vegetable that becomes enhanced when roasted in the oven with a light coat of olive oil. Butternut squash is recommended for this recipe, though any variety of squash can be used as desired. To roast the squash, preheat the oven to 350 degrees, and line a small or medium baking dish with parchment paper, then coat with olive oil. Slice the squash in half, placing each half face down on the paper and bake for approximately 35-45 minutes, until the inside of the vegetable is tender. Remove from the oven and scoop out the seeds. Place the seeds in a separate bowl, which can be used to roast for snacking. Scoop out the flesh of both halves and add to a medium bowl.

- 1 squash, roasted, seeds removed, and flesh scooped into a bowl
- ½ small onion, diced
- 4 cloves of garlic, crushed
- 1 tablespoon of olive oil
- 1 teaspoon of sea salt
- 1 teaspoon of nutmeg
- 1 teaspoon of black pepper
- 4 cups of vegetable broth

In a large cooking pot, add olive oil, onions, and garlic, and simmer on medium-low for 5-6 minutes. Add in the spices and squash, cooking for another 2-3 minutes, then pour in the vegetable broth. Reduce to simmer and cook for 10-15 minutes, stirring to combine all ingredients. Remove from the stove and cool for 15-20 minutes, then blend in a food processor in batches, until all ingredients are smooth. Return to the cooking pot and reheat, then serve.

A bowl of butternut squash soup is excellent as a meal on its own, and can also be served with a dollop of vegan sour cream. Fresh sprigs of parsley or cilantro can be added as a topping or garnish, and they also provide a boost of flavor and nutrients. Toasted squash seeds can also be prepared and added as a topping.

Cream of Broccoli Soup

Cream of broccoli soup is well-loved by many and can be recreated in the same way without dairy. Vegan butter, non-dairy milk, and other ingredients make this delicious soup possible, and it's fairly easy to create as a plant-based dish. Fresh broccoli is recommended, though frozen can be used as well. Where broccoli is unavailable, you may consider using cauliflower as a substitute by simply replacing the same portion in this recipe.

- 6 cups of broccoli florets, chopped into small pieces
- ¼ cups of finely chopped carrots
- ¼ cups of diced onions
- ¼ cups of finely chopped celery stalks
- 3 cloves of garlic, crushed
- ¼ cup vegan butter (or olive oil)
- ¼ cup of shredded vegan cheese
- 4 cups of vegetable broth
- 5 teaspoons of flour (whole wheat, all-purpose flour)
- 2 cups of almond or soy milk (unsweetened and unflavored)
- ½ cup of coconut milk (unsweetened and unflavored)
- 1 teaspoon of lemon juice
- 1 teaspoon of black pepper
- 1 teaspoon of sea salt

Add the vegan butter to a medium saucepan, and heat on medium, then add in the carrots, onions, garlic, and celery. Saute for approximately 5-6 minutes, then add in the flour, coating evenly, and cooking for a few more minutes. Slowly stir in the vegetable broth, while continuing to stir carefully and gently. Pour just a little at a time, leaving a few seconds or up to a minute in between portions. This will ensure that your vegetables are evenly cooked and mixed into the broth. Once all the broth is poured into the saucepan, add in the non-dairy milk, starting with almond or soy milk, then coconut milk, then add in the broccoli and any additional vegetables. Add the black pepper, lemon juice, sea salt, and continue to cook until broccoli is tender, then remove and set aside to cool. Blend the soup in batches, to create the creamy, thick broccoli soup texture, then return to the stovetop and reheat, stirring to cook evenly. Serve topped with shredded vegan cheese.

Lentil and Barley Soup

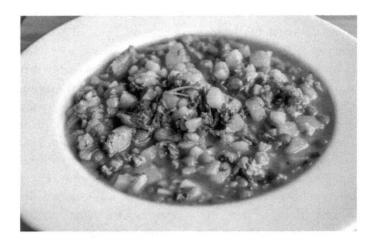

Before embracing the vegan diet, you may have enjoyed a bowl of beef stew with barley every now and then. The same type of meal can be created with a wealth of taste and nutrients using lentils in place of beef with the same barley and vegetables. This is an excellent dish to add spices, seasoning, and a variety of flavors to enhance the mild combination of lentils and barley.

- 4-6 cups of vegetable broth
- ¾ cups of lentils
- ¾ cups of barley
- 2 carrots, chopped
- 2 celery stalks, diced
- ¼ cup of frozen spinach

- 1 teaspoon of black pepper
- 1 teaspoon of sea salt
- 1 teaspoon of turmeric
- 1 teaspoon of thyme
- 3-4 bay leaves
- 1 teaspoon of dried basil leaves
- 1 cup of chopped potatoes or yams
- 2 cloves of garlic, crushed
- ½ small onion, diced
- 1 tablespoon of olive oil

In a large saucepan, heat the olive oil and add in the garlic and onion, sauteing for a few minutes. Then add in all the spices, simmering for two minutes, then add in the broth, lentils, and barley. Cook on medium-low for 20 minutes, then add in the vegetables. Continue to cook until all ingredients are tender, then serve.

Homemade Vegetable Broth

Creating a homemade vegetable broth is an excellent way to make use of vegetable peelings, skins, slices, and other leftovers that would normally be added to the compost. Fortunately, there are many nutrients contained in the stems, skins, and peelings of vegetables, including the parts we never use, such as garlic and onion skin, carrot stems, and potato peelings. These items and many others are prime ingredients for a flavorful, delicious broth, which can be enjoyed on its own or as a base for creating your own soups and stews. For the ingredients below, portion sizes are not given because the amount and availability of each depends on your own kitchen. You may add all or some of the below options, and you can combine more vegetable rinds not listed below.

- Potato peelings (make sure they are washed and scrubbed before using)
- Carrot stems, shreddings, and peelings
- Celery peelings, stems
- Leftover spinach leaves
- Cabbage leaves and stems
- Beetroot stems, including skins
- Rutabaga stems and skins, peeled
- Leftover broccoli and/or cauliflower florets, stems, and leaves
- Onion peelings and skins
- Garlic peelings and skins
- Dried herbs, such as sage, thyme, tarragon, basil, paprika, and any flavors or spices desired
- Dried bay leaves
- Sea salt
- Black pepper
- Okra stems
- Chili peppers, fresh or crushed
- 6-8 cups of water

Pour 6-8 cups of water into a large cooking pot and add all the above ingredients, starting with the spices, herbs, onion, and garlic skins. Bring to a boil and cook on high for 20 minutes, and then add the remaining ingredients. If the water doesn't cover all the ingredients, add a small amount, then cover and boil for another 30 minutes. Reduce to simmer or low heat and continue to stew for 1-2 hours. Test taste the broth and until you achieve the desired strength, then drain and use the broth as a base or as a mild, light soup on its own. Broth provides numerous nutrients on its own and can help refuel your body after a strenuous workout.

Light Lunches and Dinners

During the week, it's important to eat regular meals to ensure you're getting the most out of them, and more importantly, to determine when it is best for you to organize your training/workout in conjunction with your meals. Before you schedule your meals, becoming familiar with the various types of foods and simple preparation techniques will save you time and effort.

Avocado Wrap

Avocados are an important ingredient to include in as many meals as possible. They are rich in nutrients, such as healthy fats and fiber, and low in carbohydrates. They are also tasty and can be adapted to fit a variety of meals, from sushi rolls and dips to wraps and sandwiches. When choosing an avocado for a sandwich or wrap, it's best to use a freshly ripe option, before it becomes too mushy. Once they are easier to mash, avocados are excellent for guacamole, dressings, and other dips.

This wrap uses a whole grain flatbread with a handful of tasty ingredients to compliment the mild flavor of avocado and fresh greens with a few spices.

- 1 avocado, peeled, pitted, and sliced
- 1 cup of fresh sprouts
- 1 cup of fresh spinach leaves or arugula
- 1 teaspoon mustard
- Dash of black pepper
- 1 large whole grain tortilla or flatbread
- Smoked or seasoned (cooked) tofu

Place the tortilla or flatbread on a plate and add mustard, followed by the avocado slices, tofu, sprouts, and greens. Season with black pepper and sea salt, then wrap and serve.

Tofu and Vegetable Stir-fry

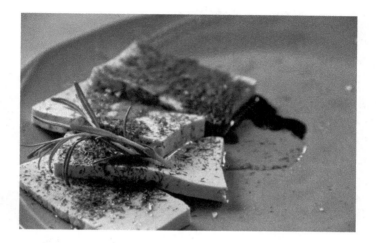

This meal is an excellent way to make use of your leftover vegetables, spices, and tofu, and it's cooked entirely in one skillet. Extra-firm tofu is the best variety for this dish and should be plain and unflavored. If the tofu was previously cooked it can be used as-is, or marinated for two hours to soak in the flavors before adding into the skillet.

- 1 block of extra-firm tofu
- ¼ cup of sesame oil
- 4 tablespoons of soy sauce

Combine the sesame oil and soy sauce into a bowl and whisk together until well mixed. Drain and rinse one block of tofu, slice into large pieces, then transfer to a resealable container. Pour the sesame oil and soy sauce mixture over the tofu, coating evenly, then refrigerate for a minimum of two hours. Drain the tofu and retain three tablespoons for the skillet.

To prepare the skillet, heat with olive oil, then toss in the tofu and leftover sesame oil and soy sauce mix. Sear on high for two minutes, then reduce to medium and continue to saute. Add in the following ingredients:

- Baby corn (five or six)
- Celery, sliced into half-inch pieces
- Half a small onion, diced
- 2 cloves of crushed garlic
- 1 chili pepper, crushed
- 1 carrot stick, chopped
- ¼ cup of snow peas
- ½ cup of broccoli, cauliflower or a combination of both
- Mushrooms, sliced
- 2 teaspoons of sesame seeds

Begin adding the garlic, onion, and chili pepper, continuing to simmer for 4-5 minutes, then add the vegetables and stir well, cooking for another ten minutes, then serve sprinkled with sesame seeds.

Lentil Dal

A popular dish in Asia, lentil dal is a simple, mild and tasty dish that is created with just a handful of lentils, spices, and vegetable broth. Lentils are an excellent source of vitamins, protein, and fiber.

- 1 cup of lentils (red, green, or brown)
- 3 cups of vegetable broth
- 2 teaspoons of sea salt
- 1 teaspoon of black pepper
- 2 teaspoons of turmeric
- ½ small onion, thinly sliced
- 1 teaspoon of cumin
- 1 teaspoon of chili powder
- 1 tablespoon of olive oil

This recipe adds a hint of spice with chili powder and cumin. To prepare the dal, heat the olive oil in a large saucepan and add in the onion, cumin, turmeric, sea salt, and black pepper. Saute for 2-3 minutes, then add in the broth and lentils. Stir regularly and reduce heat on medium. Continue to cook until the lentils are tender. Add more spices if desired, and stew for a few more minutes, then serve.

Chapter 4: Four Week Guide to Adapting to a Plant-based Diet

Are you ready to begin a plant-based diet? It's easier than you think, and it is best done with a plan to ensure you stay on track. You'll want to start with a shopping list that covers the essentials for your four-week plan. To begin creating your first vegan shopping list, determine which foods you want to buy and how you will use them in your daily meal and snack preparation. Begin by choosing which types of food you prefer according to the different categories for each nutrient:

Fiber	Protein	Vitamins & Antioxidants	Iron & Calcium	Healthy Fats
Carrots, celery, snow peas	Tofu, tempeh, miso and soy food products including cheese, non-dairy milk, and yogurt	Strawberries, raspberries, blueberries, blackberries, gooseberries, cherries	Beetroot	Almonds, cashews, pine nuts, sesame seeds, flax and hemp seeds, pistachios, peanuts
Apples, pomegranate, all berries, oranges, avocados	Almonds, hemp seeds, flax seeds, cashews, pralines, macadamia nuts, chia seeds	Apples, rhubarb, pomegranates	Spinach, arugula, broccoli, kale, parsley	Olive oil, coconut oil, grapeseed oil
Chia seeds	Kale, spinach	Oranges, lime, lemon, grapefruit	Lentils, oats, barley	Avocados

Choosing a diet high in alkaline-based foods is preferred over acidic options, which are often dairy and meat-based. Our diet should contain a higher level of alkaline-based foods, which basically covers all vegan and plant-based options. By eliminating meat and dairy, your diet automatically becomes more balanced and anti-inflammatory. While all vegan foods contain decent amounts of alkaline, some options are higher in alkaline than others. Which foods are best to choose for maximizing the benefits of alkaline-based foods?

- Olives and olive oil are an excellent option and can be added to your diet on a daily basis. They are rich in omega 3 and 6s.
- Avocados are not only a great source of healthy fats, they are also high in fiber and alkaline.
- Dark leafy greens are one of the best sources for alkaline foods. They contain many other nutrients as well, such as iron, calcium, antioxidants, and fiber.
- Lentils and beans are a great alkaline based food that provides a strong source of protein as well,

Week 1: Beginner Vegan Diet Recipes and Exercise Plan

In the beginning, it's best to follow simple recipes and ideas that are easy to cook. Choose plant-based foods that you enjoy currently, such as fresh apples, oranges, carrots combined for a snack. You can also try a simple handful of various nuts and seeds as a quick snack. You can develop your own meal plan by combining new recipes with your own favorites, which will make the transition easier to enjoy and follow. As an athlete, it's important to carefully choose the types of food and nutrients you eat in preparation for your workouts and to allow a meal afterward that replenishes your nutrients.

Start with a simple meal, such as a smoothie with added protein, like hemp, nut butter and/or chia seeds. Enjoy some simple recipes for each meal of the day, and try some new concoctions on your own based on meals you may have tried before or something completely new. The following weekly plan focuses on recipes provided in chapters two through four, while adding in some simple recipe ideas, a few of which are listed below. For your first week, focus on building a foundation of healthy foods that you will take into consideration for all of your meals: tofu, rice, beans, fruits, vegetables, non-dairy milk, and any foods that you plan to use on a regular basis.

Day	Breakfast	Lunch	Dinner	Snack/dessert
Mon	Tofu scramble	Avocado toast	Tofu and vegetable stir fry	Apple
Tues	Peanut butter and jelly smoothie	Hummus and vegetable wrap	Rice pilaf	Banana
Wed	Avocado smoothie	Roasted eggplant sandwich	Miso soup with rye bread	Hummus and crackers and/or with fresh vegetables
Thurs	Hot cereal (oatmeal with maple syrup)	Ramen noodle soup	Crepe with fried plantain and hemp protein	Coconut cultured yogurt
Fri	Pumpkin spice smoothie	Smoked tofu and sprouts wrap	Baked tempeh with sesame seeds	Rice pudding (with coconut milk)
Sat	Pistachio and mango smoothie	Hummus and veggie wrap	Leftover rice pudding with crushed peanuts, other nuts, and fresh fruit (can be served with tempeh or tofu)	Tangerines or oranges
Sun	Banana and berries smoothie	Crepes with almond butter and maple syrup	Arugula salad with fried or pan seared tofu	Peach, mango, or any fruit option

Tofu Scramble

If you're a fan of scrambled eggs, this dish will give you the pleasure of enjoying a similar taste the vegan way. Extra-firm tofu is used for this dish by marinating overnight in vegetable broth, turmeric, sea salt, and a variety of spices as desired. The following morning, tofu is mashed and sauteed on the stovetop, much like eggs, then served on its own or with toast, fresh vegetables, and/or fruit.

- 1 block of extra-firm tofu
- 2 cups of vegetable broth
- 1 teaspoon of sea salt
- 1 teaspoon of turmeric
- 1 tablespoon of olive or avocado oil
- 1 teaspoon of black pepper
- Dash of paprika
- Dash of chili pepper (optional)

Remove the extra-firm tofu from the package, then drain and rinse. In a sealable container, add the tofu, sliced into chunks (one or two-inch pieces). In a small bowl, pour the vegetable broth and stir in the spices until thoroughly mixed, then pour over the tofu. Refrigerate for a minimum of three hours, or prepare at night and marinate overnight.

To prepare the breakfast, heat a skillet on medium with olive oil. Drain the marinated tofu and retain two tablespoons of liquid. In a small bowl, mash the tofu and add into the heated skillet, then pour in the liquid and spices. Continue to saute on medium until the tofu is golden-yellow, then serve with toast, sliced avocado and/or fresh fruit.

If you want to add more flavor and ingredient options, consider spinach leaves (fresh leaves on the side or frozen, cooked spinach mixed into the tofu while scrambling), onions, sliced mushrooms, bell peppers, and other greens or vegetables leftover from a leftover stir fry.

Hot Oatmeal

A hearty and warm meal, oats are an ideal grain for breakfast as they provide fiber, iron, and protein. Oats take a while to digest, which makes you feel fuller longer.

- 2 cups of non-dairy milk
- ½ cup of oats
- 2 tablespoons chia seeds
- 1 teaspoon of cinnamon
- 1 teaspoon of low carb sweetener

In a medium saucepan, add two cups of non-dairy milk and heat on medium, adding in the remaining ingredients while stirring them. Over a period of 10-15 minutes, the oatmeal will thicken. Remove from heat when all the ingredients are tender and cooked, and pour into bowls to serve. Top with a light dusting of cinnamon and/or drizzle with maple syrup. Crushed pistachios, peanuts, or sliced almonds are an excellent addition to this dish. Coconut cream or a non-dairy milk may also be used as a topping.

Vegetable Stir-Fry With Rice

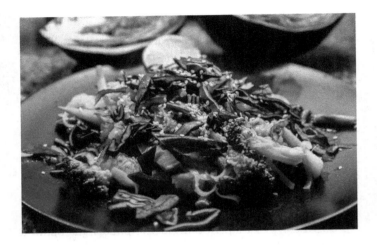

Rice is a staple food in many countries and societies, often serving as the foundation for many dishes and pilafs. Cooked rice is great as an added source of energy in salads, soups, and stews. In this dish, cooked rice is combined with a handful of ingredients in a skillet to create a fried rice dish. The vegetables are diced into very small pieces so they can mix well with the rice.

- 2 cups of cooked rice (long-grain, jasmine, or basmati rice are good options)
- 3 teaspoons of soy sauce
- 1 teaspoon of sesame seeds
- 1 carrot stick, diced finely
- 1 celery stalk, diced finely

- ¼ cup of thinly sliced mushrooms
- ½ small white onion
- 2 cloves of garlic, crushed
- 1 cup of broccoli, diced
- 2 teaspoons of olive oil

Heat a skillet on medium and add olive oil, onion, and garlic. Saute for a few minutes, then add in the finely chopped carrots, celery, broccoli, and soy sauce, cooking for 4-5 minutes until tender. Stir in the cooked rice and sesame seeds, gently folding the ingredients together to ensure all the rice is cooked and coated with the vegetable, oil, and soy sauce combination. Cook for 10-12 minutes on medium-low, then serve.

Chana Masala

Chickpeas are the feature of this dish, which combines a handful of spices and aromatic vegetables, including onions and garlic. These ingredients are stewed slowly in crushed tomatoes and spices, until softened.

- 1 can of drained and rinsed chickpeas
- 2 cups of diced tomatoes
- 1 teaspoon of cumin
- 1 teaspoon of chili pepper
- ½ teaspoon of sea salt
- 1 teaspoon of garam masala
- 1 teaspoon of curry powder
- 1 teaspoon of black pepper

- 1 tablespoon of olive oil
- 2 cloves of garlic, crushed
- ½ small onion, diced

Heat a large skillet with olive oil and toss in the cumin, sea salt, chili pepper, garam masala, curry, black pepper, garlic, and onions. Saute for 3-4 minutes, then pour in the chickpeas, cooking for 5-6 minutes. Pour in the diced tomatoes and continue to stew for 45-50 minutes on low or simmer. Serve in bowls, on a bed of rice or with flatbread.

Week 2: Implementing a Routine

After the first week of a completely vegan diet, you may notice a few changes. This can take longer depending on each individual's progress and how well you follow vegan recipes and adapt to plant-based foods. After following the first week's diet plan, it's important to plan an exercise routine in addition to and in accordance with your eating habits. This will help you plan when you eat before and after your workouts while maintaining a good handle on portion control and keeping your meal plans as easy and effortless as possible.

Getting into shape and furthering your athletic goals is a great way to stay fit and remain in good shape for many years, well into middle age and advanced age. Planning your workouts around your meals doesn't have to be difficult or detailed. You can simply choose when to "refuel" or start your "before workout" snack, usually a half-hour in advance, and plan your "after workout" food or meal to commence about one hour following exercise. The following schedule or plan is an example of how you may implement both your diet and exercise routine.

Monday

6:00 am - Breakfast smoothie

6:30-7:15 am - Cardio workout

8:00 am - Small mid-morning meal

8:30 am-12:00 pm - Work/school routine

12:00-12:30 pm - Lunch break

2:00 pm - Midday snack

4:00 pm - Leave work or school for home

4:15 pm - Before workout snack (kale chips)

4:45-6:00 pm - Workout: cardio or weights (or both)

6:15 pm - Dinner or post-workout snack (light meal)

7:00-10:00 pm - This period may include relaxation, yoga, meditation, and/or further exercise

Prepare tofu for breakfast the following morning.

Tuesday

6:00 am - Tofu scramble

6:30-7:15 am - Cardio workout

8:00 am - Small mid-morning meal (fresh fruit)

8:30 am-12:00 pm - Work/school routine

12:00-12:30 pm - Lunch break

2:00 pm - Midday snack (fruit salad and/or chia pudding)

4:00 pm - Leave work or school for home

4:15 pm - Before workout snack

4:45-6:00pm - Workout: cardio or weights (or both)

6:15 pm - Dinner or post-workout snack (light meal)

7:00-10:00 pm - This period may include relaxation, yoga, meditation, and/or further exercise

Wednesday

6:00 am - Breakfast smoothie

6:30-7:15 am - Cardio workout

8:00 am - Small mid-morning meal

8:30 am-12:00 pm - Work/school routine

12:00-12:30 pm - Lunch break

2:00 pm - Midday snack

4:00 pm - Leave work or school for home

4:15 pm - Before workout snack

4:45-6:00 pm - Workout: cardio or weights (or both)

6:15 pm - Dinner or post-workout snack (light meal)

7:00-10:00 pm - This period may include relaxation, yoga, meditation, and/or further exercise

Thursday

6:00 am - Peanut butter and toast, with fresh berries

6:30-7:15 am - Cardio workout

8:00 am - Small mid-morning meal

8:30 am-12:00 pm - Work/school routine

12:00-12:30 pm - Lunch break

2:00 pm - Midday snack

4:00 pm - Leave work or school for home

4:15 pm - Before workout snack (roasted squash seeds)

4:45-6:00 pm - Workout: cardio or weights (or both)

6:15 pm - Dinner or post-workout snack (miso soup)

7:00-10:00 pm - This period may include relaxation, yoga, meditation, and/or further exercise

Friday

6:00 am - Breakfast smoothie

6:30-7:15 am - Cardio workout

8:00 am - Small mid-morning meal

8:30 am-12:00 pm - Work/school routine

12:00-12:30 pm - Lunch break

2:00 pm - Midday snack

4:00 pm - Leave work or school for home

4:15 pm - Before workout snack

4:45-6:00 pm - Workout: cardio or weights (or both)

6:15 pm - Dinner or post-workout snack (light meal)

7:00-10:00 pm - This period may include relaxation, yoga, meditation and/or further exercise

Saturday

6:00 am - Breakfast smoothie

6:30-7:15 am - Yoga/Pilates

8:00 am - Small mid-morning meal

12:00 - 5:00 pm - If Saturday is a day off from work or school, consider trying an outdoor activity, such as cycling, jogging, hiking, or swimming.

6:15 pm - Dinner or post-workout snack (light meal)

7:00-10:00 pm - This period may include relaxation, yoga, meditation, and/or further exercise

Sunday

6:00 am - Breakfast smoothie

6:30-7:15 am - Yoga/Pilates

8:00 am - Small mid-morning meal

12:00 - 4:00 pm

During this day, try either a high-impact or moderate approach to exercise. You may want to take a break as a "rest" day. Going for a walk or treating yourself to day trip out of town are good examples of how to spend your day off, whether it's on a Sunday or another day during the week.

4:15 pm - Before workout snack

4:45-6:00 pm - Workout: cardio, weights, or a rest day

6:15 pm - Dinner or post-workout snack (light meal)

7:00-10:00 pm - This period may include relaxation, yoga, meditation, and/or further exercise

Exercises for a Healthy Lifestyle

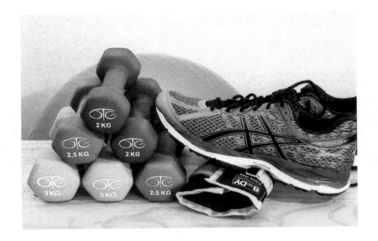

Whether you are a seasoned athlete, moderately active, or ready to get into shape, an exercise routine is the best way to get the most out of a plant-based diet. It's important to give yourself a regular routine and set goals or milestones to help you focus on self-improvement and results. To begin, try a variety of different exercises and determine what works best for you. Always keep in mind the importance of incorporating different forms of movement. This will help you develop your entire body and improve your strength, agility, posture, and endurance.

Exercise is a powerful way to stay in shape and reduce the risk of many medical conditions. It's a great way to reduce anxiety, stress, and can help people who suffer from depression. Getting active releases endorphins, which gives you a "high" that can become a regular occurrence when you workout often. There are many ways to get in shape, and while some people are partial to fast, energetic, and high-intensity workouts, others may prefer a slower pace or a strong finish with endurance. Working towards your fitness goals should be about more than losing weight. It's one of the top ways to prevent osteoporosis and similar bone and joint diseases that can occur with age.

Cardio

Also known as cardiovascular exercise, cardio is a vigorous, high impact workout that can incorporate many types of exercises or can focus just on one. These exercises are meant to increase blood flow and burn calories quickly. Cycling, running, jogging, and aerobics classes are examples of cardio.

Weight Lifting

Gaining popularity in recent years, more women and people of all ages have embraced this form of exercise as a great way to stay in shape and develop muscle. Weight training is often done at your own pace and should be, as it is a sport which it is best to start carefully. At any age, you can start with just a small amount of weights, working your way to your desired level and maintaining it for years. Weight training is an excellent goal-oriented way to improve your body's overall strength and endurance.

Swimming and Cycling

These lower impact forms of exercise are great during the summer months to explore the outdoors and get a better overall physique. Both swimming and cycling offer a full-body workout and makeover, which works well for every body type. They both help you slim down, while at the same time, help build muscle and strength.

Yoga and Pilates

Yoga is a great way to improve balance, strength, and agility while giving you a chance to relax. It's a popular way to reduce stress while helping you improve blood circulation and overall calmness. Yoga is often available at most gyms and recreation centers. If you don't have the time to take classes, there are plenty of online videos and instructions that guide you from one pose to another.

As you become familiar with the basics of yoga, you may want to explore specific styles and methods that work best for you personally. More moderate to advanced levels can be attempted at studios specifically designed for yoga and meditation.

Pilates is another excellent way to stretch and develop endurance in the body. It helps you build strength in the core of your body, which is often a struggle for many people. A regular schedule of just 15-20 minutes of pilates each day can make a significant improvement in the way you feel and in your body's condition. It can support you in other goals as well, such as in preparing for other forms of exercise.

Martial Arts

If you enjoy challenging yourself in a healthy competitive way, martial arts is a good skill to learn at all ages. Many people who study various types of martial arts are vegan or adhere to a diet that closely resembles a plant-based diet. It's a great way to develop your entire body while learning balance and improving strength, flexibility, and agility. Many community centers offer classes during the week and weekends, and just like yoga and pilates, there are classes for all skill levels.

<u>Team Sports</u>

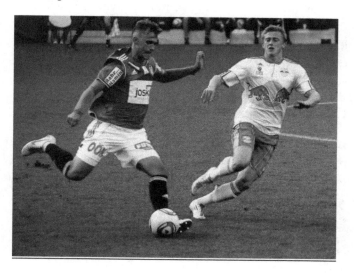

If you enjoy socializing and working as a team, baseball, basketball, hockey, and other team sports are a great option. It's important to find the right game that you enjoy most. For some people with a competitive spirit, hockey is a good option. For others, there are many clubs and groups to join to determine exactly what works best for you, whether it's outdoor baseball or tennis, or something completely different. Getting together with friends is a great way to find out what activities you enjoy doing together.

HIIT (High Impact Interval Training)

A relatively new method of exercise, HIIT aims to accomplish a lot within a short period of time. A typical workout consists of an obstacle course-like series of activities, all of them high impact and short-term, anywhere from thirty seconds to two minutes. Examples include skipping rope, lifting kettlebells, pushups, or sprinting. One rotation may consist of four or more activities, which allow for a quick rest period in between, usually one minute or less. Just one half-hour or forty-five-minute session of HIIT can equal close to the positive effects of two hours of long endurance training or similar forms of exercise.

Equipment for Exercise

Exercise balls, kettlebells, light weights, mats, and skipping rope are all excellent and inexpensive props and equipment to have for your workout. Clothing doesn't have to be specialized, as long as the fabric is comfortable and fits well so that your body can have a good range of motion.

Some people experience challenges with mobility and the ability to participate in certain types of sports and activities. Fortunately, many local clubs and community places offer modified equipment and support for this purpose. Finding an exercise partner or someone who can encourage and mentor you is an excellent way to stay motivated and keep going, even when things get difficult.

If you are new to exercising regularly and need guidance on a personal level, it's always best to check with a doctor to determine what you are able to handle. For example, if you have respiratory issues, you may need to progress slowly and not overdo yourself. If you've recovered for physical injury, don't rush into high impact exercise, even if you think it's your current level of fitness. In doing so, you may cause more damage and interfere with important healing processes at work in your body.

Week 3: Adding New Recipes

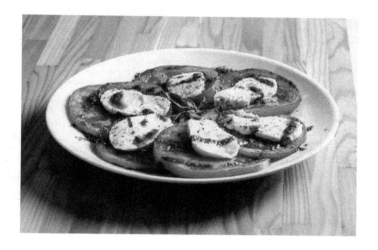

Adding new recipes is an exciting way to explore and expand your diet. Take the time to find what works best for your palate, including innovative ideas that incorporate common foods into new ideas and meals that work best for you. If you have extra time during the week or on weekends, you may want to try elaborate casseroles and baked options to enhance your plant-based meal options. On the other hand, you can also keep it simple and try as many easy recipes as possible, which can make your grocery shopping trips more predictable and easier to manage. When you encounter a new food or idea, research a few recipes beforehand so that you can become familiar with what's available to you and how to use them in a meal.

Day	Breakfast	Lunch	Dinner	Snack/dessert
Mon	Tofu scramble with spinach	Rye toast with tomato, basil leaves	Vegetable fried rice soup	Bananas
Tues	Chia seed pudding with pistachios	Beetroot hummus dip and flatbread	Miso ramen soup	Roasted squash seeds
Wed	Banana and berries smoothie	Hummus and veggie wrap with smoked tofu	Curried jackfruit and rice	Kale chips
Thurs	Tahini and chocolate energy bar	Butternut squash soup	Baked tofu with curried cabbage	Toasted red pepper and basil on flatbread
Fri	Oatmeal with coconut milk and cinnamon	Lentil and barley soup	Cream of broccoli soup	Toast with almond butter
Sat	Peaches and banana smoothie	Spinach, blueberry and almond salad	Chana masala	Coconut cultured yogurt with maple syrup
Sun	Tahini maple syrup smoothie	Roasted eggplant and cauliflower	Leftover cauliflower, chickpeas sautéed with garlic and spinach	Chia seed pudding with sliced mango

Pulled "Pork" Jackfruit

Jackfruit has become a popular fixture in vegan cuisine, making it an excellent meat replacement for pork and roast recipes. The texture of jackfruit is favorable for these meatless meals, while providing a significant amount of nutrients in each meal they are incorporated into. Most people don't realize how tasty a plate of curried jackfruit or "jerk chicken" jackfruit is without trying it. This fruit can be found canned in some grocery stores. Try one can at first, to experience the taste and potential, if you're not sure how much you will enjoy it.

- 1 tablespoon of olive oil
- 2 cans of jackfruit, drained and rinsed
- 1 teaspoon of paprika
- 1 teaspoon of chili powder
- 1 small onion, diced
- ¼ cup of tomato paste or puree
- 2 tablespoons of raw sugar
- 3 tablespoons of maple syrup
- 3 tablespoons of apple cider vinegar
- 1 teaspoon of spicy mustard

Canned jackfruit is recommended for this recipe because if fresh is used, it can be difficult and time-consuming to work with and prepare. For this reason, try canned if you are unfamiliar with this food and are using it for the first time.

To prepare this dish, drain and rinse the two cans of jackfruit in a colander, then break apart the flesh with your hands until the pieces resemble pulled pork. Heat a skillet on medium with olive oil, toss in diced onions, and saute for a few minutes. Add in the spices and tomato paste or puree, mixing thoroughly for two minutes, then add in the jackfruit, cooking until fully coated and ready to serve.

Chia Seed Pudding With Pistachios and Dried Fruits

Chia seed pudding is a delicious dessert and breakfast option, as it contains a number of energy-boosting nutrients, which can be great for a pre-workout meal or snack. Adding pistachios and dried fruits are a great option and increase both the fiber and protein levels in this dish.

- ½ cup of chia seeds
- 1 cup of coconut milk
- ¼ cup of coconut cream
- 2 teaspoons of raw sugar or maple syrup (or low carb sweetener)
- 3 tablespoons of crushed pistachio nuts
- 1 cup of dried fruits (any variety)

Combine the milk, cream, raw sugar or sweetener, chia seeds, and dried fruits together and mix well. Refrigerate for at least two hours, then serve topped with pistachios.

Aside from trying new recipes, you may want to try new cooking and preparation techniques with familiar foods. There are many vegetables, for example, that seem fairly ordinary and bland until they are incorporated into a wider range of options.

Broccoli and Cauliflower

These cruciferous vegetables are tasty on their own but are often not used to their full potential. These vegetables can be baked, sauteed, steamed, or enjoyed on their own. As an alternative to rice, they are now offered shredded or "riced" so they can be cooked and enjoyed as rice or a grain.

Parsnips

A cousin of the carrot, these tasty vegetables are often hidden in soups or stews, though they can be enjoyed raw or as part of a stir fry. Sliced and simmered on a skillet, parsnips have a very aromatic taste that is easy to enjoy.

Radishes

Pungent when they are raw, as some might enjoy them, radishes become mild and easy to digest when they are baked in the oven. They can be roasted with brussels sprouts, yams, turnips, and other root vegetables.

Turnips

A great source of vitamins and fiber, turnips are filling and make a great addition to many different meals. Often, turnips are enjoyed as a side dish, roasted alongside other vegetables or on their own. They can also be used as a substitute for potatoes if you are looking to reduce overall carbohydrate intake. There are some great, simple recipes to consider for these tasty vegetables, also known as rutabaga:

Mashed Turnips With Garlic

Turnips are pungent to taste when they are raw, though they become mellow in flavor once baked in the oven or roasted on the stovetop. They contain many essential vitamins, such as vitamin K, A, C, several B vitamins (B1, B3, B5, and B6), potassium, iron, and copper. Once they are softened, they can be easily mashed like potatoes with a variety of seasonings and/or spices, as desired.

- 3 rutabaga or turnips (small or medium in size)
- 2 cloves of garlic (whole)
- 1 tablespoon of vegan butter
- ⅛ cup of soy or almond milk (unsweetened, unflavored)
- 1 teaspoon of dill
- 1 teaspoon of black pepper
- ½ teaspoon of sea salt
- 3-4 cups of water

Bring a pot of water to boil. Peel and slice the turnips, then cut them into 1-inch pieces, and add them to the water. Add in the whole garlic cloves to cook with the turnips. Cook on high for 20 minutes, then reduce to medium, cover, and continue to cook for another 15-20 minutes, or until the turnips are tender. Drain the turnips carefully, and add both the boiled turnips and garlic cloves to a large bowl, then mash with the vegan butter and non-dairy milk. Continue to mash until all ingredients are smooth, then add in the black pepper, sea salt and dill, and serve.

This dish works well as a side, or it can be enjoyed on its own as a light meal. For a twist, add in carrots or parsnips to boil and mash for a slightly different taste.

Turnip Hash Browns

An ideal recipe for breakfast or for a snack, these can be created as a patty or in loose, shredded pieces sauteed on the stovetop. Turnips are peeled, shredded, and cooked in a skillet with olive oil. They are created much like potato hash browns. To create hash brown patties, the shredded vegetable is combined with a few ingredients in a bowl as follows:

- 2 teaspoons of olive oil
- 1 large or 2 small turnips or rutabaga
- 1 teaspoon of sea salt
- 1 teaspoon of black pepper
- 2 teaspoons of whole wheat flour

Slice the turnips and cut into 2 or 3-inch chunks. Over a large bowl, using a grater, shred each vegetable so the shreddings fall into the bowl, making about 2 cups. Add in the sea salt, black pepper, olive oil, and whole wheat flour and mix. Heat a skillet on medium with olive oil. Form into small patties or balls, about two inches wide, then add to the pan. Using a spatula, gently flatten the ball into a pattie and cook on both sides for about 3-4 minutes until golden, then serve.

Week 4: Preparing Ahead for a Future With a Vegan Lifestyle and Diet

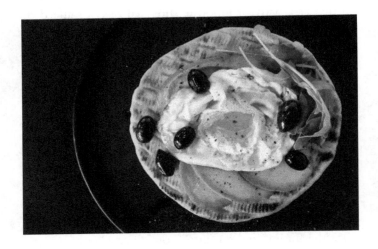

Preparing your meals and planning ahead is easier than you think. In fact, you can prepare certain foods and meals ahead of time to make the process effortless and easy, allowing you to enjoy your meals quickly. Smoothies, chia seed puddings prepared the night before, and leftover skillet dishes and stir-fries are excellent options for meals. You can also prepare food in advance by slicing vegetables and fruits, for example, to make dinner preparation easier as well.

Changing what you eat and how you prepare your food is part of it while becoming familiar with an active, health-conscious way of life is another major component of the new way you eat and live. Along the way, we may encounter some challenges that can seem like barriers until we learn to overcome them and/or find an alternative solution. The following scenarios and suggestions will help you prepare and work around these obstacles.

- Sometimes family and/or friends are not quick to support a vegan diet and may consider our move towards a plant-based diet harmful, especially if they lack the knowledge and education needed to understand it. Educating them can help, as well as giving them samples of our meals if they are open to trying them. It can take time to gain their support, but in time, anything is possible

- Find someone who is interested in the same dietary goals, whether it's a friend, co-worker, or family member. This way, it's easier to explore and enjoy all the vegan possibilities and have someone to share and discuss them with. You can track each other's progress, share advice, and encourage each other as well.

- Share new recipes at family and other events so they have a chance to enjoy them and provide feedback. Some people are surprised by how plant-based dishes can be tasty and satisfying beyond their expectations. It can ignite interest in others and give you the chance to introduce them to more vegan options.

- Don't get discouraged. If you find adapting to a vegan diet difficult at first, this could be due to changing your habits too quickly and not giving yourself enough time to adjust. This can lead to falling back on old, bad habits and forfeiting your progress.

- Give yourself time and talk to family and friends in advance so they know what to expect. This will impact the grocery list and the types of foods you will be including in your diet.

Making plans for a vegan future can take more time and preparation in the beginning, while you are still learning about and trying to understand all the new options available to you. This includes getting the most out of exploring your options before making significant changes so that you know exactly what to look for.

Chapter 5: What to Expect After the Four Week Plan

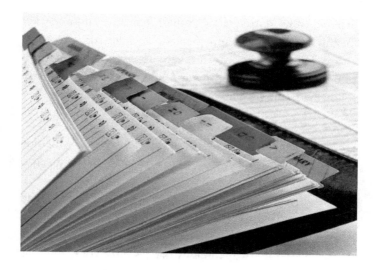

After the first four weeks of your plant-based diet, how do you feel and how would you describe your overall well-being? There are a few changes you may notice during these four weeks as a result of adapting to a plant-based diet, which includes the elimination of all dairy and meat. When you begin to see changes, some of them will be positive, while others are a bit challenging and hard to handle. It's important to realize that making a major dietary change, even if gradually or in stages, will have an impact on how your body feels.

Side Effects and Changes to Your Body

Adapting to a plant-based diet may be a shock at first, especially if you make sudden changes instead of gradually transitioning from animal-based to vegan. Some people may experience more frequency in their regularity and a quicker metabolism sooner than expected. To help adapt to these changes, drink plenty of water and eat food that is as fresh as possible. What symptoms can you expect to experience following the first four weeks of a plant-based diet?

- You'll feel more energy and less fatigue.
- Weight loss is almost always a result of switching from a diet heavy in animal-based foods to a vegan lifestyle
- Your body may become much more regular than expected, at least initially, though don't be concerned as this will settle and become less extreme over time. Chances are your body is adjusting quickly and getting rid of excess weight at the same time, both of which are beneficial.
- Your complexion may either become clear or you may break out during the early stages of a vegan diet. This is to be expected, especially when your body is detoxifying and you're suddenly eating foods that are much healthier for you than before. Over a period of a few weeks, you'll notice an improvement as your body adjusts to better eating habits.
- For many people with a diet high in processed foods, a switch to plant-based eating may come as a shock to the body and trigger a state of detoxification. This can cause some unpleasant symptoms, such as skin rashes and breakouts,

cramps and indigestion, bloating and some minor headaches. This is your body's way of reacting to change. After a few weeks, these signs will fade away, and you'll feel refreshed, with a renewed sense of energy.

Living With Changes to Your Diet

Eliminating all meat and dairy from your diet is easier for some people and more challenges for others. You may want to try making these changes to your diet in stages so that you don't feel overwhelmed with having to change too much at once. This is especially important if you live a busy lifestyle, including working full-time, raising a family, frequent traveling, and/or other commitments that require a lot of work. Changing your eating habits during this time can be challenging.

The following options can be considered as in-between stages in your transition from an omnivorous diet to plant-based eating:

- Pescatarian is a diet that is vegetarian with the exception of eating fish. This is a good step for people looking to eliminate most meat products from their diet, without making the complete switch to veganism at once. Some pescatarians may include dairy foods in their diet, and some do not.
- Lacto vegetarian refers to a plant-based diet plus dairy. People following this way of eating avoid all

91

meat products and may be selective with the type of dairy products they choose to eat as well, opting for organic options without artificial flavor

- Ovo vegetarians include eggs in their diet, in addition to a plant-based diet. They may or may not include some dairy.
- Lacto ovo vegetarians include both dairy and eggs in their diet while avoiding all meat products.

There are other forms of stages in between that eliminate just one meat and/or dairy food product at a time. It's important to choose what works best for you. If, after years of vegan living, you find that you have returned to your previous eating habits, you can always start again by using one of the above stages as a new starting point to get your plant-based diet back on track.

How to Adapt for Long-term Benefits and Lifestyle

For many people, veganism is more than a diet. It's a lifestyle change that continues for many years, possibly for a lifetime. Getting used to eating a wide variety of plant-based foods combines routine, lifestyle changes, and a different perspective on how we choose the foods we eat. This requires more than simply choosing foods that do not contain animal products or byproducts, it includes a variety of foods and expanding our discussions about food. While many people view veganism or plant-based eating as restrictive, chances are their animal-based diet centers around a limited number of meats, dairy products, and vegetables. In fact, many food items in a standard North American diet are processed and prepackaged foods, which have little or no nutritional value. Going vegan means focusing on a new world of possibility that includes unlimited options to expand what and how you eat.

Taking a Different Approach to How We Eat

When we consider all the plant-based foods available, we might initially stick only with the fruits and vegetables we like or are familiar with. While this is a good start, it's beneficial to expand our experience beyond the familiar by exploring new and different foods. How can we explore food in a fun, exciting new way with a plant-based diet?

- Look for anything new or freshly in season. Local foods that are currently in season are your best value and are tastier than their imported counterparts. If you choose imported fruits and/or vegetables, make sure you have a recipe or plan in mind to prevent them from going to waste.
- Focus on pairing the plant-based foods you like with the nutrients you need in your diet. This works wonders on prioritizing both your health and your favorite foods, which can help you get the most out of your diet and recipes.
- Try a variety of different foods and expand your regular group of options to include more fruits, vegetables, nuts, and seeds. You may be surprised

how delicious soy and vegan or non-dairy milk, cheese, and yogurt are.

- Keep a positive attitude about the change to veganism, even if it seems challenging at first. For most people, it is a major adjustment that doesn't work overnight. You may encounter comments or myths about your choice in diet, including opposing views to your own. Don't allow this to stop your progress, and continue as usual.

- If you feel concerned about the nutrient levels in plant-based foods and want to make sure you're choosing enough of what you need, it's relatively easy to research your daily requirements and make sure you get the most out of your meals in terms of both taste and nutrients.

- Many of our old choices may have centered around animal-based foods, where vegetables and fruits were served as side dishes without much thought. As children, we may have been told to eat our vegetables. However, instead of enjoying a wide range of options, many diets are limited to a small group of food options.

Always be open to change and embrace the new information and ideas you learn about to get the most out of a vegan diet.

Foods to Avoid and Habits to Change or Improve for Success

Foods to Avoid

Once you become accustomed to a plant-based lifestyle, it's important to avoid foods that will hinder your progress as an athlete and your active, healthy lifestyle. While most people are keen on eliminating meat and dairy foods for a cleaner, vegan diet, some processed and unhealthy foods may creep back into your eating habits. Sometimes, these culprits are not very obvious because they appear nutritious and balanced. Some of these foods may be found in natural food stores, where you might not expect to find unhealthy options.

Natural Candy Bars

It may seem like the lesser evil when choosing a snack, especially if there are no animal products and the label states "all-natural". Unfortunately, these treats might contain hidden sugars and food coloring that may not appear as an obvious ingredient on the wrapper or container. Some candy bars with natural flavors and ingredients may also have artificial contents which are combined to look and taste natural. For this reason, it's best to avoid all candy bars, even those pretending to be organic, made with real fruit, and low in sugar because often this is inaccurate.

Chemically Dried Fruit

Dried fruits make excellent, healthy snacks provided they are naturally sun-dried. Unfortunately, many dried fruits are prepared using chemicals, which can decrease their nutritional value. Always look for "sun-dried" when choosing dried apricots, raisins, prunes, and berries. Naturally dried fruits are not chemically altered and will retain many of their beneficial nutrients.

Vegetable and Fruit Chips

These snacks may seem like the ideal alternative to potato chips and pretzels, though they can be just as unhealthy or inaccurately labeled as natural. While it is possible to create natural vegan chips, many store-bought varieties are not as high quality as they claim. Often, they contain added sugar, sodium, and/or artificial ingredients to boost the taste.

Canned Vegetables (With Exceptions)

While canned beans and legumes are often the handiest and most convenient options available, it's best to avoid canned vegetables that can otherwise be found fresh or frozen, such as carrots, broccoli, green beans, asparagus, and celery. Your best option for the most nutrient power is fresh, then frozen, followed by dried or canned. Most grocery stores and food markets feature their local, in-season options. Buying in season, indigenous produce is the very best of all your options and will reduce the amount of greenhouse gas emissions because they are locally available.

Pastries and Baked Goods

With the exception of whole grain bread and similar foods, it's best to skip pastries and cakes altogether. Even where all-natural ingredients are used, they are full of processed grains, sugars, and flavors without any nutritional value. For this reason, they should be avoided and replaced with energy bars and similar treats that are homemade.

While some packaged foods may seem like a good option sometimes, it's good practice to avoid any foods with a hefty list of ingredients and additives. These can become addictive and harmful in the long term.

Any Foods or Desserts With Gelatin

Gelatin is a pork-based product and should be avoided. It can hide inside a number of pre-packed desserts and foods, such as jello and pudding.

Some Alcoholic Beverages

Egg products are often used in the making of beer and wine. Some of the brewing processes include using animal-based products as well. As an alternative, there are vegan options for wine and beer available, which may be in a local store or specialty shop.

Pasta and Noodles

Most varieties of pasta contain eggs, though there are rice noodles and egg-free varieties available. Check the ingredients to be certain. Most stores will also carry gluten-free options as well.

There are a lot of hidden and unexpected ways animal-products can wind up in your grocery basket, even when you are trying to stick to vegan options only:

- Some produce contains a wax coating that can contain animal byproducts as an ingredient. Avoid fruits and vegetables with this coating, and always rinse and peel the skins of foods that may be suspect of this wax. If you buy from a local grocer or farmer's market, it will be easier to avoid

- You may already avoid milk chocolate due to its dairy component, though some dark chocolate varieties have trace amounts of dairy or milk products as well. It's important to read labels to avoid them. Fortunately, most dark chocolate products are vegan, and some are labeled as such for clarification.

- Potato chips and other vegetable chips may seem like an enjoyable snack now and again, though they should be avoided for two reasons: they are highly processed with chemicals and often contain traces of dairy, specifically cheese in their flavoring.

- Deep-fried foods should always be avoided, even if they are vegan. There is often a chance they have been fried alongside meat products, which can transfer easily.

- Bone char, which is derived from cattle, can be found in some refined sugars. It's best to avoid sugar as much as possible and substitute with maple syrup, low carb natural sweeteners, or raw sugar options. Coconut sugar is another option to consider.

- Some non-dairy products are not 100% dairy-free and should be carefully reviewed to ensure they are compatible with a plant-based diet.

- If you enjoy beans and prefer to buy them in a can, always avoid flavored options that may contain lard or pork products. Some beans are prepared with a tomato-flavored syrup that may seem vegan initially but can contain trace amounts of pork.

It's always best to check the labels and research your products before you buy them. It may only take a few minutes to learn something new that will improve your diet and make shopping a rewarding learning experience. (A. Petre, MS RD, 2016)

High Nutrient or "Superfood" Options

When you choose your foods, you may want to consider the following superfoods, which are rich in a variety of nutrients and help close the gap on the potential for deficiencies.

Chia Seeds

Popular in low carb puddings, hot cereals, and smoothies, chia seeds are full of nutrients and can often provide the requirements you need with just a small amount. Chia seeds provide iron, calcium, fiber, omega 3 and 6s, and antioxidants. They are versatile and easy to include in your diet in many different ways.

Berries

Strawberries, blueberries, raspberries, blackberries, and cherries are all excellent sources of fiber and antioxidants. They are easy to enjoy on their own as a snack or breakfast. Fresh or frozen, berries are a great way to boost the nutrient content in your diet without much effort.

Avocado

A natural fat source and a good source of fiber and vitamins, avocados are excellent on toast, with eggs, in smoothies, or in a variety of other dishes, including sushi and salads.

Kale

Kale is a bitter vegetable that combines well with other flavors, such as sweet and spicy, to give variety to the taste. Kale, like other dark green vegetables, is very high in nutrients, while it has an added bonus as well. Kale includes calcium, protein, iron, fiber, antioxidants, and vitamins C and A. Eating kale regularly, as part of a smoothie or salad, can improve your health greatly and help prevent a number of diseases.

Almonds, Hazelnuts, Walnuts, and Pecans

Basically, all nuts are considered high in nutrients and an excellent way to get the healthy fats, protein, and fiber you need every day. They make a great snack and can be mixed with dried fruits for a trail mix.

Tips for Shopping Vegan

When you start shopping vegan, you'll notice a lot of products cater to the plant-based lifestyle. The produce aisles and frozen food sections will become familiar territory after a while, as you'll do most of your shopping in these areas. It's important to avoid overspending too much on items that are trivial and overpriced due to a brand name or popularity attached to it. While you may enjoy a vegan burger now and again, the store-bought variety can be expensive and an alternative can be easily made at home. When you create your first plant-based shopping list, you may want to consider the following:

- Stay within a reasonable budget by avoiding pre-packaged foods, even if they are vegan and look delicious. They can be added as an option once you have all the main or staple foods chosen.

- Make fresh and/or frozen produce a priority because these foods are often reasonable in price and contain most of the required ingredients you need every day. Frozen vegetables, berries, and other produce are ideal for keeping longer, and the nutrients are just the same as in the fresh option.

- If you used to shop for meat and dairy, visit the dairy alternative section of your local grocery store to get familiar with these products. For example, there is probably a coconut-cultured yogurt that contains a lot of the same nutrients as the milk or dairy counterpart. Vegan cheese is often vegetable or soy-based and can make an excellent topping for many dishes.

- Buy and cook in bulk. This will save you money in the long run. If you have a large freezer, you can create meals at least one week in advance. This allows you to avoid needing to buy and cook more often during the week, when you might be most busy. Buying in bulk should be considered carefully, as some stores will charge around the same for certain products, even in bulk, than others. You may find that certain products are more expensive than others, regardless of whether they are in bulk or not. It's important to research and factor in the math before making decisions about these foods.

- Eating at home may not always be available to you, though it can be one of the best ways to save money and avoid overpriced meals out. Some restaurants and eateries, looking to "cash in" on the vegan lifestyle, charge more for certain vegan meals due to their popularity. Many people enjoy a plant-based meal prepared by a chef or skilled cook, though making it at home can seem like a lot of work and not worth their time. Fortunately, there are many great recipes online that can give you either elaborate or simple versions of every recipe you've ever wanted to try, all without animal products.

- Include whole grains in your diet, and avoid box cereals and processed goods as much as possible. This will ensure you skip the high fructose corn syrup and high amounts of sugars often found in box cereals. If you eat processed cereal every day, removing it as an option can make a profound difference in just a couple of weeks.

- If you have a grocery store with free samples, always check if there is a vegan sample and/or product available, if the food item is of interest. Many food brands now include vegan options for everything, as more people than ever are sticking to a vegan diet.

- If you have other dietary needs, such as low sugar and/or low carb eating, there are plenty of plant-based options for these as well. A low carb diet is another emerging way of eating, and as veganism grows in popularity, many people will make the strategic choice to combine both a plant-based and low carb diet.

In general, don't make your grocery shopping trip a stressful event. Keep it simple, and don't be afraid to try new foods and options that fit well into the vegan diet. Once you have a basic or template shopping list ready, you'll have a much easier time factoring in all the requirements.

Chapter 6: Frequently Asked Questions

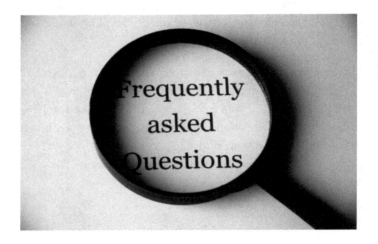

Once you embrace a vegan diet, you'll continue to enjoy the many benefits of living a plant-based lifestyle along with all health improvements and support needed for an active lifestyle. Adapting to a vegan or plant-based diet is different for everyone, and while some people switch quickly and have little or no difficulty making the change, others may bounce back and forth between ways of eating. There is no right or wrong way for everyone, as dietary and health choices are an individual's decision. The following frequently asked questions can help you satisfy your curiosity about eating and living a plant-based lifestyle.

Question: Do vegans often switch back to animal-based eating when plant-based options don't work anymore?

Answer: Firstly, a plant-based diet will have varying results for everyone, and while it's an ideal way to live and eat, there are some challenges to overcome. For example, people with an iron deficiency or the need for higher levels of certain nutrients should have their needs assessed by a medical professional to determine with nutrients they need more of. For iron, dark greens and beetroot are excellent options and should become a regular part of your diet.

Question: Is eating too much soy or soy-based foods dangerous?

Answer: Some people are allergic to soy or soy-based foods, and these individuals should be sure to avoid soy products. For people with soy allergies, choosing nut-based milk and other vegan substitutes are a growing option. For others with a sensitive stomach, eating a lot of soy can cause some digestive discomfort. In some situations, fermented soy foods, such as miso and tempeh, are easier to digest and don't contribute to bloating, as regular soy products can. For most, soy is a healthy food that can be included as a regular part of a vegan diet.

Question: Is it more expensive to eat plant-based food, and if so, how can it be affordable?

Answer: Any diet or way of eating can be expensive if you choose organic, imported, or specialty foods, including artisan food products that cost a premium. There are a few options to reduce the cost of food when shopping vegan:

- Choose only local produce at small grocers and independent businesses. They are more likely to give you a discount on your grocery bill or a better deal for your money.

- Buying in bulk is a good option and can save you a lot of money, especially if you buy large quantities of specific items, such as beans, rice, chia seeds, and other various seeds and nuts.
- Buy in season when fruits and vegetables are less expensive.

Question: I made the mistake of eating animal products after a successful switch to eating vegan. How can I get back on track?

Answer: Firstly, don't feel guilty about your experience and realize that this happens to everyone. Most people will "slip" and have a meat or dairy-based food item. If it happens just once or twice, you can simply jump back into plant-based eating without any issues. Depending on how long you were vegan, you may notice some indigestion as your body is no longer accustomed to animal-based foods. If you change back to eating meat and dairy has continued for some time, you can either gradually reintroduce yourself back into veganism or switch back completely, depending on your comfort level.

Question: How do I know if a plant-based diet is improving my health? What are the signs I should watch for?

Answer: What to expect during a switch from a traditional diet to plant-based eating varies for everyone. Unfortunately, when some people suspect it isn't working they quit too soon and forfeit any benefit they may have gained. In fact, many benefits go unnoticed because they are not frequently tested. This includes lower blood pressure, healthy insulin and glucose levels, and many other advantages. Unless you regularly monitor and notice changes, it can be challenging to realize if anything is happening. For some people, it can take months before a difference such as weight loss or other benefits are obvious, which can cause friends and family to question why you choose vegan eating. If you feel discouraged, just remember that the goal is not short-term or temporary, rather, it is a long-term solution with many reasons to continue, even in the face of criticism.

Question: Is it acceptable to raise my children on a vegan diet?

Answer: Yes, absolutely, though special care should be taken to ensure they get all the nutrients and benefits of veganism possible. This is especially important for young children, for whom it may be best to consult a medical professional or registered dietician to make sure your kids, like yourself, get balanced meals that cover all their daily nutrient requirements. Supplement where you suspect or find a lack of certain vitamins such as B12 or vitamin D. If you are ever in doubt, consult a medical professional for advice.

Another point to consider when thinking about children and vegan eating is this: giving your children the option to choose whether or not they want a vegan or animal-based diet.

Question: Are there any health conditions or other reasons that would render a plant-based diet unacceptable for someone?

Answer: Fortunately, everyone can adapt to veganism, and when there is a condition that causes a severe deficiency, it can most likely be resolved with supplements and/or eating enough foods with this nutrient. For example, iron deficiency anemia can be easily remedied with sufficient amounts of iron. If you're not getting enough by eating beetroots, spinach, and kale, then taking a daily supplement will keep your iron at a healthy level.

Other deficiencies that may arise for some people on a vegan diet include vitamin B12, vitamin D, protein and/or calcium, however, this is only the case if you don't eat a wide variety of food with the various nutrients requirements. It's important to keep in mind that deficiencies and a lack of nutrition can occur in any diet, especially when you don't take the time to determine the best options available. Many people eat limited amounts of vitamins before they go vegan, and when they do, their habits must change as well.

Question: Are non-dairy versions of dairy and meat products healthy? It seems that some of them may be processed and can cause more harm than good.

Answer: Non-dairy products vary in quality and ingredients, where some are completely soy-free and vegetable-based, while others are soy-based. If you have allergies to soy, there are often non-soy options available, and if you are concerned about the ingredients used to make them, it's important to read the nutrient labels and research which brands and/or companies are best. For example, you may want to buy your soy-based foods from a local source that provides organic products.

Question: Is it risky to be vegan when you are pregnant or breastfeeding?

Answer: Often, people will go off and back on a vegan diet, and when there is a major life change, they will either start or return to a plant-based diet, or the complete opposite. As with any other situation, veganism is a healthy and sustainable way to eat during pregnancy. The most important goal during pregnancy is making sure you keep all of your nutrient levels, including your proteins and iron, in a healthy range. This can be done by eating only plant-based foods, though you may choose to supplement if it becomes an easier option. Regular checkups with a medical professional can help you determine if you should supplement or make any changes.

Question: My family and/or partner isn't interested in or supportive of going vegan. How can I continue without their support, and will it be more difficult?

Answer: There will definitely be challenges that come with eating vegan while living with someone who isn't, especially if they eat very differently. This can be more costly when grocery shopping as well, as adding those vegan options to the cart may be seen as an extra item for a diet that your partner doesn't participate in. Instead of doubling the effort, try to negotiate by asking your partner which vegan or plant-based foods they enjoy. You'll be surprised how many they can choose, as most people enjoy fresh fruit and vegetables. Your partner may be pleasantly surprised by how tasty some vegan versions of their meat and dairy foods can be! If some products are too expensive, there are plenty of homemade vegan burger recipes, for example, that can involve portobello mushrooms or create patties from various beans, spices, and whole grain ingredients.

Sometimes, all it takes is an open mind for someone to understand the positivity of a vegan diet and what it can bring to many people's lives. For many people, going plant-based is one of the best ways to slow down or reverse medical conditions that would otherwise become debilitating. For others, it's a fresh start to a new way of eating that can make them feel younger and more energetic than ever before. For these reasons, a plant-based diet can become a long-term way to live.

Question: Where are the best places to shop for vegan food options?

Answer: You can shop anywhere! Veganism is popular and plant-based foods are everywhere, including some of the most general, bare-bones grocery stores. You'll notice tofu and soy products in most, if not all, grocery stores. If you are concerned about the quality of your food in addition to eating vegan, try shopping at local markets and ordering from farms who deliver or offer a similar service. Small, local, environmentally conscious organizations are often linked to vegan or plant-based advocacy groups, which can direct you towards good places to find high-quality foods.

Question: I need support but my family and friends are not vegan. Are there any support groups for athletes and vegans or both?

Answer: There are many vegan and plant-based groups offering support, information, and education about veganism. They may host events where cooking shows and demonstrations, including food samples, are made available. You may find some cafes that offer and support meat alternatives, and some may offer a menu that is completely vegan. If you are finding it difficult to implement plant-based eating into your life because of time constraints and not having the support available, there are food delivery

110

options and online support groups that can satisfy both of these needs.

Online support groups, recipe ideas, and forums are a great way to meet others going vegan and to discuss any concerns you might have. People are eager to participate online because they can remain anonymous, and most people are supportive and positive on these sites. In some forums, there are a lot of shared opinions and advice from people who have been vegan for many years. This makes the process easier to follow and more enjoyable. You might find several new uses or ideas for common foods that you wouldn't have otherwise considered.

Question: Since weight loss is a major benefit of a plant-based diet, is there a guarantee that I will keep the weight off as long as I remain vegan?

Answer: There is no complete guarantee, though the chances are in your favor if you stick with healthy, whole foods and avoid processed, high sugar foods as much as possible. The purpose of a plant-based diet is twofold: to follow a diet based on eliminating all animal-based foods, and to choose the right foods that are nutrient-rich and support your health. As long as you maintain a balanced diet without excessive sugar and artificial ingredients, you can safely avoid weight gain and maintain your current weight.

Question: How can I introduce a plant-based diet to other people?

Answer: The best approach to introducing a vegan or plant-based diet to family and friends is by example. Offer them a serving of one of your creations or post a vegan recipe on social media. Some people will give it a try and possibly give you their feedback as well.

The journey to a plant-based lifestyle is one of the most important decisions you'll make in life and one that will provide a lot of advantages in the long-term.

Question: How is veganism more sustainable?

Answer: The more people rely on plant-based foods and products, the less feed is needed to raise animals for this purpose. This reduces the space and resources needed to raise animals because they are no longer farmed or are farmed in fewer numbers. If this shift would occur en masse, you would notice less carbon emissions and less energy used. This is a more sustainable way of living because it takes more energy to farm animals and the crops they eat than to farm crops for our consumption alone.

Question: Many celebrities, including professional athletes, are vegan. It seems they are more open about plant-based eating than ever before. Is there a reason why it's more popular now?

Answer: There are a few reasons why plant-based eating is more popular now than ever. Celebrity endorsement is definitely helping promote veganism, and people from all backgrounds are enjoying a diet that is meat and dairy-free. In the past, a lot of people associated vegetarians and vegans with a rare or specialized type of diet, whereas today it's mainstream. Here are some of the reasons why:

- It's well known and researched that plant-based eating will maintain a healthy body weight. People who follow a vegan diet are leaner, more energetic, and are likely to never become obese.

- As the movement towards an animal-free diet grew, more people tried it as a "fad" diet, though the effects are long-term and the health benefits are significant. Over time, it becomes more of a lifestyle than a diet, which can set a healthier standard of living, as well as eating, for years to come.

- Awareness about cruelty to animals and avoiding cosmetics that test their products on animals is another reason why many people now embrace veganism. While some activism may appear extreme, with demonstrations and campaigns, in general, people tend to view animals as sentient beings, deserving of care and respect. For this reason, many people have become cautious about the amount of meat in their diet.

- People who have suffered cardiac arrest, strokes, and other cardiovascular complications have found major success after going vegan. Not only do they improve their chances of good health and longer life, but they also lose weight and feel better too.

Question: Do you metabolize and break down plant-based nutrients better or more quickly than meat or dairy?

Answer: Yes, in fact, for this reason, you'll notice a faster metabolism and improved regularity within a short period after starting a vegan diet. This is due to the high fiber content in fruits and vegetables. Also, plant-based nutrients are simply easier to digest and transport through the blood, which means their use is more effective than animal-based nutrients that take longer to metabolize.

Question: Is every vegan an activist for animal rights?

Answer: Activism is important to create awareness for animals, however, most people who follow a plant-based diet simply do just that. The majority of people who eat vegan may not appear obvious at all, and you may be shocked to find out when it's a co-worker or friend. While a lot of people choose this way of eating for ethical reasons, they may not choose the path of activism but simply choose their food options wisely and live as an example instead.

Question: Is it best to consume more grains and foods rich in carbohydrates before a vigorous workout?

Answer: Both yes and no apply here because it depends on your personal goals and how much energy you need. If you've already reached your fitness and weight goals, you could benefit from additional energy to fuel marathons and cross country skiing, cycling, and swimming. For short-term workouts and weight loss targeting, you may want to make better use of your own energy in the form of stored calories to achieve results.

When and if you add carbohydrates to your diet, choose nutrient-rich options such as quinoa, oats, barley, and other whole grains. Avoid processed, high sugar options that don't give you any nutritional value beyond just the carbs. Protein is important as well, though eating more than you burn means your body will need to find storage, and this can defeat your goals and the purpose of exercise.

Question: Is there a model plan or template for a workout and eating schedule, or should this be modified to suit individual needs?

Answer: Everyone has a different schedule with a variety of commitments and events they need to prioritize. Your health and fitness are priorities too, and they can fit into many different scenarios, whether you are a stay at home parent, work days or shift work, or change your plans often. The plans and schedules in this book are a guide and foundation for your own custom plan. Getting the most out of your diet means striving for balance and making sure that your lifestyle will help you reduce stress and stay healthy, content, and productive.

There is no one-size-fits-all plan for everybody. Each person has a goal or set of goals they want or need to achieve. Combining fitness and veganism is a great way to take you there. It's never too late to start, nor is it too difficult to continue and follow once you begin.

Always remember to start and work towards your goals on your terms. This is of great value and your health is of utmost importance. Take as much information and education as you can from various resources, such as workshops, cooking classes, recipes, and if possible, a few classes with a personal trainer, to help you start your routine on the right foot. Along the way, you'll learn a lot from your own mistakes, which is something positive that can drive you to achieve more next time. Getting the most out of a plant-based lifestyle means striving for more and better. You owe it to yourself to utilize the benefits of health and wellness to enjoy life and get the most out of it.

Conclusion

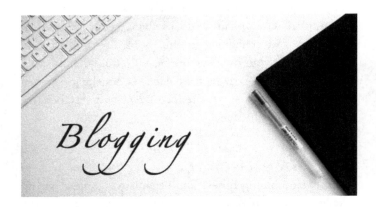

Choosing a vegan diet is a wonderful way to improve your diet and support an active lifestyle. You can greatly improve many aspects of your life and take the time to explore many different foods and options for plant-based eating as you embark on your journey.

Tips and Suggestions

Getting started on a vegan journey and taking steps to achieve this goal is different for everyone. It's important to understand that everyone will have a different experience, and this includes athletes and people with all levels of fitness. The following tips and suggestions are a general guideline to help you remain focused and motivated every step of the way:

- If you fall back on old eating habits, don't be hard on yourself. Everyone has a different approach towards going vegan, and circumstances can change for anyone at any time. Give yourself recognition for making positive dietary changes and focus on moving forward, instead of on your mistakes.

- Give yourself time to adjust to plant-based eating, and don't rush into any change unless it is well thought out. It's never ideal to rush into change, especially when it's a major overhaul of your current eating habits. Your body will adapt more easily if you make changes slowly, step by step

- Don't skip a product because it looks unappealing at first. You may be pleasantly surprised by the amount of healthy, tasty vegan foods waiting in your local markets and grocers. While some products may be expensive, they can be a nice treat on occasion. You will also have the option of researching and comparing brand names and the quality of the product before making a firm decision. Not all products will become your favorite, though it's important to try something new every once and awhile.

- If you don't like the idea of buying non-dairy almond milk or other nut-based milks in the store, you may be interested in making your own. While this can take a bit of time and preparation, it can be a rewarding experience.

- Always read the flyers before you shop and know what you are looking for. If you wander into a store without a plan in mind, you're likely to overspend and choose the wrong foods or not what you really wanted. Establish a threshold for costs and allow for some flexibility where possible. If you're new to veganism, it can take time to figure out exactly what works best.

Transitioning Into Veganism With Family and Friends

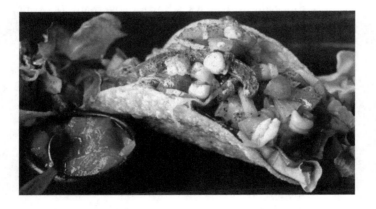

One of the most rewarding aspects of going vegan is enjoying the experience with friends and family. Sometimes, our choices influence others, and this makes it easier for them to transition as well. For most people, it's a big change, and having someone to support them and make those changes can mean a lot. This is especially rewarding when you have athletic and/or active family and friends who have the same goals as you for fitness and living well. There are some helpful tips and suggestions that can help your group succeed with a plant-based diet:

- Check your pace and the pace of your family and/or friends. Are they likely to get ahead of you in any way and if they do, are you ok with it? Some people are driven on their own and will gladly join others on their journey to veganism. This doesn't always mean that you'll progress in the same way. In fact, sometimes one person may slip back into their previous habits and re-start again, while other people make the change completely without going back. If you find that there is variability in the level of progression between you and your group, it's ok, but check in with them from time to time so that you can help motivate one another.

- Join a cooking class that features vegan cuisine. This is a great way to experiment with some new recipes and to learn about how fruits and vegetables are used in daily cooking outside of your current meal plan. A cooking class is also a fun event where you can meet other people who may have the same or similar dietary goals. You'll gain new knowledge of how to prepare food while learning new skills and making new friends.

- Don't be hard on yourself. We are all capable of making mistakes and feeling the effects of them. Life is full of choices, and sometimes we become our own worst enemy when it comes to making changes when we expect to succeed entirely without error. This level of perfectionism isn't healthy and should be swapped for a kinder, gentler way of caring for yourself. The goal of vegan eating is to support your body and health throughout your life. This will take time, and you shouldn't expect perfection at any stage during the process. There will always be room for improvement and this is acceptable.

- If you find that the process of making a lot of changes to your diet is too much at once, take a break. It's not going to happen immediately for everyone, and taking care of yourself by avoiding stress is the best plan of action. Don't force yourself to make all the changes at once, and instead, work in steps at a pace that is best for you.
- In the beginning, and even throughout your meal planning, keep it simple. Make sure you build a pantry that includes the basic spices, seasonings, and dried goods you need, and keep buying the fresh and frozen produce and foods that work well with your options.

Always give yourself plenty of time to schedule and prepare ahead for meals and exercise. In doing this, you'll find yourself in a relaxed, low-stress situation without having to prepare a meal at the last minute. Scheduling your workouts is a great way to keep yourself focused on your goals without distraction. Coordinating meals and exercise is the perfect solution for optimizing your overall health and sense of well being.

CPSIA information can be obtained
at www.ICGtesting.com
Printed in the USA
BVHW051046040121
596933BV00007B/518

9 781801 542500